THE GRADUAL VEGETARIAN
LISA TRACY

"In this book Lisa Tracy do _____ _____
She shows her readers who are concerned about too much
meat in their diets how to become vegetarians, gradually and
comfortably. Preparing meals, eating out, and dealing with
unconvinced family members are all dealt with here in a clear
manner.

At any point in the transition one can stop where one is
comfortable. If one wants to just cut out the red meats from
the diet, she shows how a balanced diet can be constructed
using eggs, chicken, and fish. If one wants to go all the way to
just veggie vegetarianism, Tracy helps one adjust slowly and,
I think, painlessly.

More evidence from the scientific literature indicates that all
of us should try to aim for vegetarianism. We need roughage.
We need less fat in the diet. We need the minerals from
plants. We need to chew.

This book would be a welcome addition to one's kitchen for
the recipes alone. Thank you, Lisa Tracy; you are helping us
do it."

—Lendon Smith,
Best-selling author of
Feed Yourself Right

"For anyone thinking about becoming a vegetarian or just
wanting to live a healthier life, Lisa Tracy's book is the one to
rely on. With step-by-step instructions, _The Gradual Vegetar-_
ian will help you change the way you live and what you eat as
much as you want. Diet is crucial for longevity and this book
is crucial for a long, healthy life."

—Steven Petrow, Senior Editor, _Longevity_

QUANTITY SALES

Most Dell books are available at special quantity discounts when purchased in bulk by corporations, organizations, or groups. Special imprints, messages, and excerpts can be produced to meet your needs. For more information, write to: Dell Publishing, 1540 Broadway, New York, NY 10036. Special Markets.

INDIVIDUAL SALES

Are there any Dell books you want but cannot find in your local stores? If so, you can order them directly from us. You can get any Dell book currently in print. For a complete up-to-date listing of our books and information on how to order, write to: Dell Readers Service, Box DR, 1540 Broadway, New York, NY 10036.

THE *Gradual Vegetarian*

LISA TRACY

A DELL BOOK

Published by
Dell Publishing
a division of
Bantam Doubleday Dell Publishing Group, Inc.
1540 Broadway
New York, New York 10036

If you purchased this book without a cover you should be aware that this book is stolen property. It was reported as "unsold and destroyed" to the publisher and neither the author nor the publisher has received any payment for this "stripped book."

This book does not substitute for the medical advice and supervision of your personal physician. No change in diet should be undertaken except under the direction of a physician.

The recipes for Basic Nut Bread and Cornell Bread are from *The World of Breads*. Copyright 1968 Dolores Casella. Used with permission of the publisher, David White, Inc., Port Washington, New York.

Copyright © 1985 by Lisa Tracy

All rights reserved. No part of this book may be reproduced or transmitted in any form or by any means, electronic or mechanical, including photocopying, recording, or by any information storage and retrieval system, without the written permission of the Publisher, except where permitted by law. For information address M. Evans and Company, Inc., New York, New York.

Designed by Ronald F. Shey

The trademark Dell® is registered in the U.S. Patent and Trademark Office.

ISBN: 0-440-21585-4

Reprinted by arrangement with M. Evans and Company, Inc.

Printed in the United States of America

July 1993

10 9 8 7 6 5 4 3 2 1

RAD

For Paul and Owen,
my dear companions

Contents

ACKNOWLEDGMENTS

The Romans had a useful phrase for it: *sine qua non,* "without which not." These paragraphs are devoted to those without whom this book would not have been possible.

Thanks to the Conlow family, who put up with it all and provided support, encouragement and recipes; to my sister, Jeanne Eichelberger, who typed, edited, and assisted in so many ways; and to my mother, who arrived at the eleventh hour to see it through.

Thanks for their special expertise to Dr. Bob Evans, professor of biology, and Dr. Spencer Knapp, professor of chemistry, Rutgers University; Terry and Susan Ingram of East West of South Jersey, and to Craig LaRoche and James Lennon of the American Natural Hygiene Society.

For a wealth of assistance and ideas, including recipes, thanks to: Robert Baum, Barbara Chilcott, Ilene Conlon, Bill Coyle, Ed Dodd, Patti Duffy, Connie Fernandez, Mary Flynn-Day, Rayetta Fossen, Susan Greatorex, Tobi Hartzell, Marie Herrmann, Meg Herron, Cheryl Hess, Virginia Sederis Hillhouse, Arnold Jackson, Kathleen Johnson, Nancy Kiessling, Carol Thompson Lajczok, Connie Langland, Katie Letcher Lyle, Sally Munger Mann, Marilynn Marter, Linda

Winters Meeh, Grant Parnagian, Nannie Poindexter, Donna Richards, Selwyn Ryba, Larry Schweers, Rebecca Sinkler, Jack Sweeney, Judith Sylk-Siegel, Nancy Szokan, Elaine Tait, Miriam Taub, Fawn and John Vrazo, Herb Wurth, Nancy Zehler.

And to Calley O'Neill and Jeanne Sharpe, for changing the way I thought about the food we eat.

Special thanks to the people at M. Evans, to copy editor Joan Whitman, and to Charlotte Sheedy and Regula Noetzli, for making the book a reality.

INTRODUCTION

In the past ten years, Americans have been doing themselves a big favor: getting healthy. We are exercising at an astonishing pace—on foot, on wheels, on water or on the ubiquitous carpeting of the health spa floor. At the same time, a change has come over our kitchens. We are trying foods we never tried before, healthy foods, and liking them.

With landmark studies by the National Institutes of Health and the American Cancer Society to back us up, we are increasingly looking for ways to cut down on fats and cholesterol. For many, this means eating fewer animal foods, and more vegetables, fruits and grains for a healthier lifestyle. It is touted in runners' magazines and sold by the week in expensive health spas, but the truth of the matter is that this is a lifestyle not only for athletes or for dieters. It is a way of eating that can be easy and rewarding for anyone. *The Gradual Vegetarian* tells you how to shop, cook and organize so that you can practice your new lifestyle successfully no matter where you are or with whom you're eating.

If you have ever thought about waging war on fatty foods —or found yourself choosing fish over meat—or paused at the vegetable bins in the supermarket over some exotic new

11

fruit or vegetable—you could be a gradual vegetarian. Most of us resist overwhelming changes in our lives, and our eating habits are no exception. The beauty of being a gradual vegetarian is that you can do it at your own pace. That's why the book is divided into stages. Stage One is for people who are ready to think about eating less meat. There are fish and chicken and a host of vegetable and dairy dishes, many of them already familiar. Stage Two is the traditional vegetarian middle of the road—vegetables and grains, eggs and dairy food. Stage Three presents an entry to the stricter vegetarian diets.

The Gradual Vegetarian offers a step-by-step guide to vegetarian dining. You may be drawn to vegetarianism for economic, moral, or health reasons, and you may decide at any stage that you have reached the level of vegetarianism that suits you.

Whatever your motives, a more vegetable-oriented diet can bring health benefits. Studies comparing vegetarians with the rest of the population in recent years have shown that cancers of the breast, colon and prostate are more common in people who eat a diet rich in animal fat; they are less common in vegetarians. Government reports have identified in meats a number of suspected carcinogens and other toxic chemicals associated with birth defects or mutations.

Weight-conscious Americans also are discovering that a vegetarian diet can be slimming. Carbohydrates were once taboo to dieters. Now the complex carbohydrates, the high fiber and the plant proteins of vegetables, fruits and grains are recommended to combat obesity as well as other health disorders.

For me, vegetarianism has been at various times a trip from Stage One to Stage Three and back again. In each stage I have found valuable techniques for healthier cooking and interesting recipes that have traveled with me. I have also discovered that healthy food for most people doesn't have to be as bland or boring as some of the diets you've tried might have you believe. It can be scintillating, exotic or hearty. You decide.

This book is intended as a guide, a reference book and a source of recipes. Vegetarian cooking doesn't have to be complicated and can be done by people of virtually any level of skill in the kitchen. And as consumers become more health conscious, the food industry is cooperating by offering a wider range of healthier foods. Fresh fruits and vegetables are available year-round, and whole grains are no longer difficult to find. In restaurants and even fast-food outlets the vegetarian diner finds a choice of suitable foods. There has never been a more convenient time to be a gradual vegetarian.

And it's guaranteed to be worth your effort.

THE
GRADUAL
VEGETARIAN

STAGE ONE

ONE

ANALYZING YOUR DIET

As American as Mom's apple pie. That's us. If it isn't, we have a sneaking feeling it ought to be. The Norman Rockwell Thanksgiving dinner is firmly ingrained in our minds as an ideal, the *real meal.*

Part of the trouble with meals is that they represent more than food. They represent companionship and our earliest notions of security, and that's why when we start trying to change our eating habits we almost immediately run into trouble. What, me give up Mom's apple pie? I'm a meat-and-potatoes man. Let's sit down and discuss this over a drink. I'll get back to you during my coffee break. All I'm really looking for is a little tea and sympathy. What's the sweetener in the deal—you know, the frosting on the cake?

Our attitudes toward food are pervasive. Everyone knows that sweet, rich, meaty and creamy are terms of praise. Who would try to advertise a meal, a piece of literature or a new fabric by describing it as bland, sour, bitter, thin or squashy? Corny is a term of opprobrium. When it comes to food, it is no exaggeration to say we have been programmed, by everyone from well-meaning parents and teachers to the food industry.

17

So the first thing to do in attempting to change is to analyze our own diet, to determine what we eat, when, and why. Have you been programmed to believe you *need* three square meals a day? Are there foods you don't like? Do you find that you accept coffee, sweets, or beer and a hot dog just because they're offered, and it's easier than saying no?

The goal is to detach ourselves, slowly if need be but persistently, from habits that don't serve us well, and cultivate those that do. Stage One is a good time to quit eating some kinds of meat; cut down on caffeine and sugar; think about quitting smoking; experiment with new styles of eating. You may be surprised to discover how many good habits you already have that you never even thought about.

Do yourself a favor and give yourself credit for whatever you're doing right. You like vegetables? Good. Seldom buy prepared foods? Great. Order cheese ravioli instead of meat, or linguine with clam sauce instead of meatballs, when you eat in an Italian restaurant? Terrific. Like fish? Eat lots of greens? Better yet. Count any and all positive habits as points in your favor. Then start planning a strategy to expand what's right about your diet.

THINKING OF CHANGING

You may have stumbled onto the information that vast quantities of meat aren't good for you. Or perhaps you've heard of Frances Moore Lappe's *Diet for a Small Planet* (Ballantine Books; 1971), in which she so cogently points out that it takes 16 pounds of grain to produce one pound of beef, grain that could just as well or better be used to feed the world's starving. Or perhaps you're just dismayed at what grocery prices are doing to your pocketbook.

Ten years ago you would have snorted if anyone had suggested that you would one day be a vegetarian. Now you're thinking you would be, if you only had time to figure it out.

There seems to be such a volume of information about balancing incomplete protein sources, and those protein sources themselves are forbiddingly esoteric in their preparation and not all that appetizing. And the time and effort involved in planning a vegetarian menu every night just isn't available to the beleaguered working parent, or the beleaguered single person who doesn't do that much cooking or eating at home anyway. To say nothing of the looks on the faces of your loved ones when you start explaining that spinach isn't a side dish. And how would you explain it to co-workers and more casual acquaintances?

It is indeed undeniably overwhelming if you try to do it all at once. Setting aside the philosophical considerations, the real reasons most people reject the idea of changing their diets are practical, and they are chiefly three: time, money and know-how.

People perceive a vegetarian cuisine as being time-consuming, and the health food store as an expensive specialty shop. And they feel they cannot afford the time or energy to learn a new style of cooking that they see as complicated and composed of unfamiliar and unappetizing ingredients.

It is true that eating differently from the mainstream of society takes an initial mental effort—that decision to take charge of our diet instead of eating or buying what's put before us. And yes, the health food store can be forbidding, but at least there is little likelihood that you are getting anything in your food but food when you shop there. And for starters, you don't even have to. If you have a good supermarket, you can start there. If you live in a neighborhood that has a fruit stand or farmers' market, so much the better.

And of course it takes time—as much time as we are willing to spend to prepare as many of our own meals as we are willing to fix. But you don't have to be a gourmet cook to master the skills involved in a vegetarian cuisine. Nobody was born knowing what to do with raw broccoli. And the point of being a gradual vegetarian is that you start from where you are.

WHERE TO START

The first vegetarians I met were in New York in the late sixties. My image of vegetarian dishes conformed to the cooked vegetables of my youth. Bland. Squashy. A little soggy here, as in spinach; a little mealy there, as in lima beans.

Of course it wasn't so. These vegetarians I met didn't lurk in the corners of restaurants over lukewarm dishes of over-cooked succotash. They dined in style on tempura and sushi, fresh salads and homemade breads. I loved the elegant simplicity of their meals. I bought a cookbook and went into culinary culture shock.

By the mid-seventies, I had figured out how to keep the rice from sticking. I had also noticed something. It was easy enough to eat vegetarian meals in the privacy of your own home with nobody around. But how often was life like that? The problem with vegetarianism, I began to think, wasn't food, but people. What I needed, I thought as I fell off the vegetarian wagon for the third time, was a plan. Then I realized—I didn't have to do it all at once. The idea of Stage One was forming in my mind.

The idea of Stage One is to assess your present eating habits, noting the ones that could be construed as vegetarian. You map out a new shopping strategy that makes better use of the supermarket, and locate some other food sources. You work some new recipes into your repertoire, and—if you need to—learn some basics. If you work or feed a working family or if you eat away from home a lot, you deal with how to avoid unhealthy foods when your kitchen isn't handy.

This works equally well for the vegetarian or would-be vegetarian who is living with a confirmed meat eater or a junk-food junkie. That's because what we are really talking about in Stage One is a middle ground that should be comfortable to people with all kinds of eating habits, as long as they're willing to try something new once in a while.

BUT WHAT ABOUT MEAT?

If you have ever looked at any diets designed for losing weight, you will have noticed that they discourage the dieter from eating pork entirely and limit his intake of red meats—notably beef and lamb—to a few times a week.

The fact that it is necessary to tell someone that he must limit his intake of red meats to several times a week implies that people are routinely eating red meat more often, perhaps many more times a week than that.

In this country in this century that may be true for people of means: middle-class and upper-class people, the ones the magazine diets are aimed at. We have been programmed to believe that terrible things will happen to you if you don't get enough protein; that it's tough to eat enough protein every day unless you really work at it; that meat is the only complete protein; and therefore that you'd better eat meat every day.

We have also been programmed to believe that because meat is largely made up of protein and contains no carbohydrates, eating meat will make you skinny, because everyone knows carbohydrates are starches and sugars and they make you fat.

Only recently have doctors and nutritionists begun to back-pedal. The picture that is now beginning to emerge is that carbohydrate sources like fruit, vegetables and grain products, the unrefined grain foods that haven't been stripped of their nutritional value, are more easily digested than meats, are virtually fat-free, and do not contain the hormones often fed to livestock to fatten them up.

Meats, on the other hand, contain mainly saturated fats—bad for you because they're hard to digest and the body can make relatively little use of them. Moreover, it turns out that meat-preserving substances like nitrites in bacon have been linked to cancer. That excess hormones are bad for you. That frying meat on metal at high temperatures can create substances called pyrogens that are also linked to cancer. And that pesticides and other toxic substances accumulate in animal tissues as they pass up the food chain.

Meat, moreover, is getting so expensive that it is becoming a luxury, not only for people at the bottom of the economy, but also for people who thought they were in the middle. The food industry's response is to offer the consumer Hamburger Helper, as if the consumer who really needs a break didn't have enough sense to figure out that he could make it cheaper at home.

The conjunction of forces in our society is making more and more people reevaluate their traditional way of eating. On the one hand there's the growing expense at the checkout counter, and meat is not an item that you can easily grow, process and store at home for yourself. On the other hand, an information explosion has made people much more conscious of their health, and new concepts of glamour have made new forms of behavior socially acceptable—even fashionable—and therefore easier to indulge in. If you had served raw vegetables at a cocktail party years ago, you would have been deemed mad or hopelessly out of it. That was when processed clam dip and do-it-yourself onion soup and sour

---

DID YOU KNOW? Carbohydrates—fruits, vegetables and unrefined grain products—are more easily digested than meat, are virtually fat free, and do not contain the hormones used to fatten livestock.

---

cream with potato chips were the life of the party. Now raw vegetables are called *crudités* and they're omnipresent.

Whatever your reasons for becoming a vegetarian, it's never too soon to contemplate reaping the fringe benefits of improved health that any conscious attention to your diet can give you.

That's why this is a good time to think about quitting smoking, if you do; to wean yourself from coffee and sugar; and to keep in mind that the simpler your preparation of food, the easier it will be for your body to digest it.

We are already putting an incredible strain on vital organs including the heart and the liver, and on the adrenal glands, just by living in a developed society in the twentieth century: with the air we breathe, the water we drink and the stress we endure driving to work, getting home, getting ahead, living in congested cities with high-crime areas or in artificial suburbs where there is little real sense of community and the automobile is the only way out. The stress makes the adrenals work overtime, throwing the body into a permanent state of high gear; the toxins we ingest must all be processed by the liver and carried away by the bloodstream. That's why anything we can do to help—even if it means quitting smoking or eating seaweed—is just plain smart.

Did I mention seaweed? Oh, but not in Stage One—not unless you're really convinced that you're going the whole route, in which case you can start slipping it into your minestrone.

THE COFFEE-TEA-MEAT-SUGAR-TOBACCO SYNDROME

These are all what Naboru Muramoto, in the system of Oriental medicine he presented in *Healing Ourselves* (Avon Books; 1973), calls extreme foods. And what you do when you ingest extreme foods is jerk your body around. You eat a meal of meat, potatoes cooked in grease or with a fatty blob of sour cream on top, maybe a cocktail or some wine. Your body signals for time out—a siesta or even hibernation. But you are planning to go back to work or you have the whole evening ahead of you. Instinctively and from long habit you know what to do. You give yourself a jolt of adrenaline by downing a cup of coffee, perhaps with some sugar. Unless you drink it black, chances are you also lace it with some nondairy creamer, made from coconut oil (saturated fat) with assorted preservatives thrown in. And if you're a smoker, you have a cigarette. The adrenals kick over and that overfull ate-too-much feeling goes away. The meat, the grease, the fats and the stimulants—coffee, sugar and nicotine—create a balance. Or, if you want to look at it another way, they are part of a vicious circle.

That's why when you start changing your diet you will actually find it easier to kick those habits. It's really not too much to do all at once: The lighter foods don't go very well with those heavy stimulants anyway. You may keep having that cup of coffee and that cigarette—but secretly you'll find they seem superfluous.

There are two other advantages to quitting now: You'll give your taste buds a break in their exploration of some new foods. And you'll have the psychological advantage of making a clean break.

I will talk more about the Oriental philosophy of balancing foods in Stage Three, when we take a look at some of the more advanced vegetarian diets. But for the time being we can understand this idea of extremes in very practical terms. The main habit we are dealing with, physically and psychologically, is eating, but the peripheral habits matter too, especially drinking, smoking and exercise. This is true in any diet. And we should think of this or any diet, not as a set of rules imposed from the outside, but as a system of our own devising, which we will tinker with until we get it to work well for us.

In this system, we know that extreme stimuli like alcohol and tobacco can distort our assessment of our eating habits, so it makes sense to limit or eliminate them in any way that works. As for exercise, it can help by improving the circulation and even changing the metabolism, the way our bodies burn the foods we give them. It also serves as a distraction from snacking. Brisk walking is something most people can do, and increasingly are doing, even during lunch breaks at work. Some people even use that time for running, changing and showering before returning to their desks. Biking and swimming are also good, since they can be done at your own pace.

So can yoga, which is very good for dealing with the daily stress of life and keeping things in perspective. It also is especially good exercise for improving blood circulation, which in turn promotes general health and helps rid the body of accumulated wastes. Yoga classes are inexpensive, and once you learn the basic postures you can do them at home.

It doesn't matter at all what kind of exercise you choose, as long as you like it well enough to stick to it. But you should make at least one kind part of your overall strategy.

WHAT'S IN IT FOR YOU

It is important to allow yourself freedom from preconceived notions of what constitutes a meal. Our culture's current ideas about that derive from the affluent post–World War II period in which the "typical" American family was supposed to have a full-time homemaker and a set of rising expectations. Among these were expectations that one's diet would reflect and broadcast one's financial status. They culminated in the arrival of gourmet cooking and all its paraphernalia as a fad in this country.

The enormous benefit from this has been to expand our ideas about eating and to make new equipment, techniques and food readily available. The drawback has been the tendency to try to keep up with those rising, trendy expectations. In today's economy and with our knowledge of the world's needs, it is important to liberate ourselves from fashions that have become exorbitant—including those notions about what constitutes a "square" meal or suitable fare for guests.

And speaking of economy, there are some trade-offs you may enjoy in cutting down on meat products and junk snack foods. You may simply find that food bills are lower. Or you may allow yourself the "luxury" of good quality in the food you buy, whether at the grocery store or the health food store —butter instead of margarine, real cheese instead of processed, better oil, exotic vegetables. Look at it as an investment—and as the break you really do deserve.

TWO

MAPPING A STRATEGY

You can start changing your eating habits at any time of the year. In the summer, there is the advantage of a wealth of fresh fruits and vegetables, and the tendency to eat lighter, which makes the idea of salads or a European lunch of cheese, fruit and bread appealing. In winter, there's the comfort of soups, stews and baked things.

Part of the ultimate vegetarian philosophy is that you eat what is native to your climate and eat it in season. This isn't our concern at present, but a good way to start your change-of-diet strategy is with a look at what's available in your supermarket.

In Stage One, we are making meals around chicken and fish, and also meatless entrées: pastas, egg and cheese dishes, vegetables and rice and legumes. The idea is to start with what is familiar, or easy, or both, and build from there. Simple baking and some desserts that avoid sugar and refined flour will be included.

You need a shopping list to get a fair idea of your current shopping (and therefore eating) habits. Start by figuring how far in advance you can reasonably plan your meals, and shop for that length of time. If you work at home, are a homemaker, or have a job with regular hours and duties, it may be easy to shop for a week at a time. If you shop for a longer period, chances are you are not relying on fresh fruits and vegetables. If you have a high-pressure job that involves a lot of running around, you don't need anyone to tell you your diet can suffer for it, and that's partly because it's next to impossible to plan ahead. Do it a little at a time.

If you work, you may want to concentrate at first on changing just one meal: dinner, because that's the one you are most likely to eat, and because you can eat it at home and control its content without anybody looking over your shoulder.

If you have a family to plan for, your task is multiplied by the number of mouths you feed and the personal tastes attached to them. Again, starting with dinners may be the simplest approach.

So start with a shopping list for what would normally feed you for a week. First notice how many and what kinds of fruits and vegetables are included—fresh, frozen or canned. Notice how much and what kind of bread you're buying; what proportion of meats to fish and dairy products and their comparative costs; how many convenience foods, snacks and prepared desserts; how much coffee, tea and sugar.

If you're not a close reader of labels, start. Read the label on every single food product you buy. By Food and Drug Administration (FDA) regulation, ingredients must be listed in order from greatest to least. On a stroll down the cereal aisle, you'll discover that sugar is the number one ingredient of several of the leading brands and the number two ingredient in most of the others, even the ones that prominently advertise themselves as "natural" or "granola." One of these, billed by its maker (a major name in cereals) as having "eight essential vitamins and iron," contains the following in order: sugar, wheat, corn syrup (more sugar), partially hydrogenated (that means heat-treated) soy oil, honey, caramel color, salt, sodium acetate, sodium ascorbate, niacinamide, reduced iron, vitamin A palmitate, lecithin, pyrodoxinehydrochloride

(B_6), riboflavin (B_2), thiamin hydrochloride (B_1), folic acid and vitamin D_2. Don't be seduced by the list of vitamins, since it is unlikely your body will assimilate much of them while absorbing this incredible dose of sugar, especially since they are not occurring in their natural form but have been added artificially to "fortify" the cereal.

If you're lucky, you may find four cereals on the aisle that contain no sugar, but you'll have to really look for them. That's because the cereals at eye level are all the giant-size boxes of sugared cereals destined for speedy consumption by people who don't know any better. The unsugared cereals are typically off to the side on a bottom shelf somewhere. They include, among cold cereals, most kinds of shredded wheat, Post Grape Nuts (but not the Grape Nut Flakes), and Quaker unprocessed bran, which is a good thing to mix in with your cereal. Compare prices and you'll be delighted to find that they cost anywhere from one-third to one-half less than their sugared counterparts with the toy offers on the box.

Also in the no-nonsense cereal category are the hot cereals. Here the major cereal companies seem to have done better in resisting the tendency to process the life out of the grain and compensate with sugar. Again read the labels. And if you haven't eaten hot oatmeal since childhood, you're in for a pleasant surprise. It's not nearly as lumpy as you remember and it tastes a lot better.

Reading labels in the canned food department may also bring a surprise or two, as you realize that virtually all canned vegetables include salt and many contain sugar as well, as do most canned fruits, of course. The second or sometimes even the first ingredient is likely to be water; so while a pound of fresh peaches may cost slightly more than a pound can of peaches, it really costs less in terms of what you get out of it, as do fresh mushrooms, potatoes, carrots—you name it. Frozen vegetables represent a better food value than canned; unfortunately, freezing really ruins the texture of most fruits and vegetables. And frozen foods are relatively expensive. On the whole, you'll get best value for your wallet and your body if you make a habit of buying fresh produce in season.

While you're shopping, this time following your normal buying habits, notice what proportion of your total grocery bill is going for meats, coffee, tea and snack foods—and for what period of time you expect each to last. Make similar note of dairy products, fresh vegetables, fruits and fruit juices, breads and cereals. Your present diet and what it costs in dollars should be emerging. Remember to give yourself credit for any good habits you may discern.

WHAT YOU EAT

Our eating habits are so deeply ingrained that there's not much chance of our developing a new diet against our will. While it's possible to learn to like to eat something that is utterly repulsive to you at first bite, you could better put the effort into learning to love five or six things that merely looked or tasted a little strange at first.

Many people, for instance, are revolted by the texture and the whole idea of tripe, yet in Italy it is considered a great delicacy. Sheep's eyes are a treat in Morocco, and the Japanese swear by raw fish. And how many times have you been told liver is good for you?

Interestingly, the hard-to-eat foods that come to mind first are all meats, perhaps because we are such meat eaters. But there are people too who find okra disgustingly slimy, or spinach bitter. Miso and seaweed do unquestionably taste strange the first few times you try them, and tofu is bland. But you can also wake up one day with a craving for them. And they *are* good for you.

But you don't need to start with miso. You start where you are. Where you are at this point is in front of the kitchen counter, putting away stuff from the supermarket. How much is canned? Packaged? Raw? Junk food? Solid? Liquid? Whole grain? Processed? Contains sugar?

Having begun to analyze your buying habits, you can also tune into your eating habits. It is important to know what you like, and your tastes can be cross-referenced according to temperature, texture, consistency, flavor and degree of saltiness and spiciness. To make any kind of a diet work for you, you need to know what you will eat, what you won't, and what you feel deprived without.

Maybe it's hot food, for instance—I mean, hot as in soup or cooked entrées. Maybe you can get through the day nibbling on raw carrots and crackers or whatever, but you really feel you *need* a hot meal at night. Or maybe you need something hot at every meal, even if it's only soup or toast. Or maybe you don't feel a meal is a meal without something sweet at the end of it, or you have an aversion to food that is squishy.

If you're a person who feels a meal isn't a meal without meat, relax. Nobody is going to take that bone away from you in Stage One. Start by eliminating one or two kinds of meat from your diet—the fatty ones, pork and lamb—or all red meat. Substitute chicken and fish. You could start with just one or two completely meatless dinners a week, as many people did easily enough when meat prices rose dramatically in the early seventies. Perhaps you do that already. Add chicken a couple of times a week, and fish once or twice. Pretty soon you've got six or seven days with no red meat, no problem.

Experiment with the composition of the menu, too. It is not written anywhere in stone that dinner consists of one helping of meat and two vegetables. Sometimes when I was starting out on this venture, I'd just have the two vegetables. Broccoli with lemon and a big baked potato with a little butter and a heap of cottage cheese or yogurt was my favorite. Coming home late from the office, I found the traditional big American dinner was not only a nuisance to fix, but also unnecessary and probably unhealthy, too, with bedtime just a few hours away.

Since the human mind is blessed with a faculty for juggling, you can be analyzing your shopping and eating habits constantly, every time the occasion arises for a coffee break, a meal out, lunch at work, or the question of whether or not to eat breakfast. And at the same time you can be experimenting with weaning yourself away from old habits and taking on new ones; testing how hard the transition seems to be; and developing new tastes.

HOW YOU EAT IT

I group possible dinner menus primarily by hot and cold (or winter and summer, if you prefer), since temperature in food seems to be important to me. I find that on all but the hottest days, I like to have something hot at night, even if it's only a cup of soup. On that basis, I might think ahead for a week of meals in summer and end up with something like this: (1) a meal of pasta and vegetables, maybe with cheese; (2) broiled fish with a couple of vegetables, or one vegetable and green salad; (3) a baked potato with cottage cheese and a vegetable, or rice with stir-fried vegetables; (4) soup, hot or cold, with green salad and some good bread; (5) a salade Niçoise—a French dish incorporating tuna and cold potato with greens and tomatoes; (6) stewed chicken; (7) leftover chicken. If you have a family of hearty eaters on your hands, soups, salads and vegetable side dishes can be good meal extenders.

In the winter a week's menu would probably rely more on soups and less on salads, with an omelet, a tuna-noodle casserole, or a vegetable casserole or quiche thrown in.

It is important to note a couple of things. First, every meal need not be a production. In fact, it better not be, or you won't do it. It's just too hard, especially if you're working. Thus, homemade bread doesn't have to mean made by you, but it should be whole-grain bread, wherever you buy it. Thus, in a pinch soup can come out of a can or package *if* you read the ingredients carefully, and a green salad doesn't have to have six different vegetables, all of which need fine slicing or a fancy dressing. And thus, none of the above meals requires gourmet skills.

Second, there are some shortcuts you should avoid:

■ If vegetables are your main course, they should be fresh and cooked from scratch with whatever personal touches you may add in the way of seasoning. That way they'll be better quality, you'll feel more at home with them, and you won't feel shortchanged of a real meal.

■ Refined white rice is a waste of time, money and energy. Minute rice I won't even discuss. Converted rice shows up well in comparisons for protein against brown rice, but is processed. You may as well learn to cook brown rice. It's not hard, it just takes a little longer. Grains ultimately are the staple that replaces meat in a vegetarian diet. Brown rice is probably the most widely used, and it's satisfying to eat and good for you.

■ If you're eating salad, you might as well get used to dressing it yourself. Again, it's not hard. It just takes a little time to do it and you can even cut that by making a big batch at a time. Or by just tossing the greens lightly with a little oil and lemon juice with salt and pepper.

■ Convenience foods as defined by marketing analysts have nothing to do with good nutrition. Whole cookbooks have been predicated on the novice's fear of tangling with real, raw, unadulterated food, the "I-hate-to-cook" and "gourmet-meal-in-10-minutes" schools of thought. But why is it any simpler to open a can of some cream soup that's heavily laced with refined flour, salt and preservatives and dump that in your tuna casserole than it is to dish a few spoonfuls of plain yogurt out of the container and mix that into the casserole with your own amount of salt, which might even be none at all? And do we have so little respect for our own survival—which is after all what food is all about—that we really want to dispense with it in 10 minutes and with absolutely no personal thought about our individual needs? When you think about it, this is precisely what the bulk of advertising has told us is so over the last several decades. But the advertisers, let's remember, are not primarily responsible for your health.

GROWTH OF A STRATEGY

As soon as you think you have a handle on your basic shopping and eating habits—it could be as soon as that first shopping list or as long as weeks, depending on how much time you put into it—start moving toward instituting any or all of the following changes:

■ Dinners built on fish, dairy food, fresh vegetables, fruit and whole grains instead of meats, convenience foods, prepackaged vegetables and prepared desserts.

■ Lunches that include fresh fruits and vegetables, whatever else they also include. If you eat lunch at work, this in itself may constitute quite a feat of ingenuity, but in an age where even Roy Rogers has a salad bar, it can't be impossible.

■ Breakfast. Nutritionists seem to agree that we eat more sensibly if we don't skip this meal, so if you're not a breakfast lover, maybe you should give it a try. Try a breakfast that doesn't include eggs as a regular thing, since you may want them as a meat substitute at other meals. Cereal is simple to fix, with pancakes or waffles as an occasional treat. Fresh or cooked fruit is a good addition as often as you can manage it. If you use fruit juice, be sure it has no added sugar.

■ Pretend you aren't a product of twentieth-century America. Explore the diets of other cultures, with or without meat. In the Orient, rice is the staple, served with whatever else is available—hence the tendency in Chinese and Japanese cuisine to serve meat in tiny bits, if at all, with vegetables over rice. What began as economic necessity among peoples all over the world, where one chicken might be expected to feed twenty people, is good practice today. If you don't think you can give up meat in one swoop, eat less and stretch it further. When I make stewed chicken, for instance, I add lots of vegetables. The big pieces of chicken get taken at the first meal. But before I put the leftovers away, I pull out all the bones, remove the remaining meat, and put it back in the pot. The chicken the second day is truly a stew, with more vegetables per person than meat.

◼ Restaurants. If you eat out, apply the same criteria. Steer your eating companions to Oriental or Indian restaurants. Is there a vegetarian restaurant nearby? Be brave. Ask for explanations and try any dishes that sound good. In regular restaurants and diners, scrutinize the menu for salads, soups and egg or fish dishes. Italian menus offer many meatless possibilities, and a good Italian restaurant will offer fresh cooked vegetables as a side dish. Don't go back to places where you find instant mashed potatoes or dishes that obviously came out of a can; it's your money. Avoid deep-fried foods; even diners usually have one broiled fish entrée, and the fat in the deep fryer is almost invariably rancid.

◼ Shopping. If you have a good supermarket, you can be a pretty successful vegetarian without recourse to the health food store, although you may not have the greatest variety of grains at your disposal, or the best quality. But for a few items you probably must go to a health food store. They are raw honey (optional), cold-processed oil (a must), and sea salt or tamari (soy) sauce. All are discussed in detail later.

THE HEALTH FOOD STORE

Once you're in the health food store, there's nothing to prevent your shopping around. For the present, virtually any health food store will do, although I would be suspicious of one that displays products like grains in open containers unless the store has a great volume of business to insure a quick turnover.

For the long run, there are certain things you will be looking for in a health food store. But for the present, it is enough just to get acquainted. Use your stop there for the cold-pressed oil as a chance to browse. Read the labels on cereals, pastas, yogurts, teas and baked goods the same way you do in the supermarket, and compare prices. Note what variety of items is available, how fresh they seem, how the store is laid out.

Typically you'll find an aisle for cereals and whole grains; an aisle of flours and pastas; a section for dried beans and peas; one for dried fruits and nuts; aisles of vitamins and cosmetics; a section for herbal teas; several shelves of oils; a book section; a section of refrigerated foods and perhaps one of frozen goods; and a section of prepared mixes, usually based on soy products, that are intended as meat substitutes.

If you have the time and energy to comparison-shop in several health food stores, you'll find that they are not all alike. Some belong to chains; others are individually owned and stocked. Some are more expensive than others, and their selection and even quality of merchandise will vary.

For many items, it probably doesn't matter whether you buy them in the supermarket or the health food store. For now, concentrate on establishing a workable routine that fits into your daily life. Shopping is as essential to your diet as cooking, and you won't do it if it's not convenient.

Speaking of convenience, please notice on those rare occasions when you visit a "convenience" store that they are practically useless in terms of food. They offer no whole wheat bread, no fresh vegetables except perhaps some iceberg lettuce and warehouse-ripened tomatoes; their yogurt has no live cultures; their cheese is processed and their cereal sugared. So much for convenience.

To sum it up, mapping a strategy is the first concrete step toward changing your eating habits. It includes an appreciation of your present diet, observation of the ways each meal can be changed, an assessment of your shopping possibilities, and a decision to make whatever changes your routine can tolerate.

The next step is to look at each meal in more detail, and to start developing a repertoire of menus that can become routine without being boring, then refine your cooking and shopping habits around them.

THREE

SHOPPING
VEGETARIAN

Our shopping list for Stage One will be built around staples, the items that don't spoil quickly, that you can keep on hand for a week or more at a time and turn into a meal with little fuss. Surprisingly, some of these are fresh vegetables.

Keeping a supply of healthful staples on hand is one of the most useful things a busy person can do to improve his or her diet. The basics are augmented with more perishable items as needed: in Stage One, more fruits and vegetables, dairy foods, chicken and fish.

Stock up on the basics about once a month, if it makes your life easier, freezing things like bread and butter. With the basics in the house, and the weekly complement of dairy foods, you will never have nothing to eat. When you do have time, you can augment the basics with spur-of-the-moment shopping for variety.

CARROTS AND ALL THAT

You are now heading down the fruit and vegetable aisle with an empty shopping cart. Always start here. It's a good habit to get into. You should always have carrots, cabbage, celery, potatoes, onions and garlic in your kitchen. Refrigerated (for cabbage, celery and carrots) or kept out of hot places, they will keep for weeks and even months, and provide you with quick and easy meals. So you never eat cabbage? Get some anyway. You'll be surprised how good it tastes in stir-fry. Fruits that keep well, though not as well as the vegetables, are apples and citrus fruits. Buy them in season. It's especially handy to have lemons around, for salad dressings and fish, or to add zest to almost any dish.

On to the cereal aisle for grains. Read the labels carefully; for instance, the granola mixes say "natural" in big letters, but they typically have sugar or other refined sweeteners in them, often as a main ingredient, and you are better off making your own, or buying it at a health food store. Buy the unsweetened cold cereals, and plain bran and wheat germ if you like; and any of the unsugared hot cereals, such as Wheatena or Quaker Oats. Admittedly most supermarket cereals contain preservatives, but it's a start. The bran provides fiber, the wheat germ valuable vitamin E, protein and oil, and the other cereals bulk and texture as well as protein, vitamins and minerals. I use the granola sparingly because it is rich and relatively expensive. Topping the cereal with fresh or cooked fruit eliminates the need for other sweeteners.

The wheat germ and bran, by the way, should be refrigerated as soon as they are opened, as should any flour. The plain rolled oats or Wheatena are good hot cereals for winter mornings, with milk and fruit or with butter and a little honey (not too often) or maple syrup. The oats are also used to make your own granola.

Next are the whole grains, dried legumes and flour. Get a

box or two of brown rice, a package of lentils, a package of split peas, and perhaps a package of barley. You are now equipped to make a variety of soups almost indefinitely and on the spur of the moment, to say nothing of rice dishes.

On to the flour. Buy a bag of unbleached, such as Ceresota, and one of whole wheat if they have it. Get a box of baking soda and a can of baking powder while you're at it. You are now ready to make delicious pancakes, muffins and quick breads from scratch. They're easy.

If you are near the pasta, pick up some spaghetti, lasagne, linguine, elbow macaroni or shells, and egg noodles. Need I say that these are the stuff of which infinite instant meals are made?

Canned goods. Stock up on a few cans of minced clams and some tuna, unless you happen to have a conscientious objection to tuna fishing practices, in which case I guess you could substitute salmon. Of the canned soups, Progresso doesn't seem to be loaded with preservatives, corn starch, flour or meat derivatives. Even here you have to read the labels, but some of the soups are okay, and are handy for emergencies, such as sick people left to fend for themselves. At this stage of the game you probably should also buy canned kidney beans and chick-peas, because dried beans take at least a couple of hours to cook, and are best if soaked overnight, and you won't always have that much time. Stock up on plain canned tomatoes, whole or puréed, for soups and sauces. You may want tomato paste as well, though a perfectly good sauce can be made without it, and it does contain sugar and lots of salt.

About the only canned fruit that doesn't contain sugar seems to be pineapple. Buy it if you like it. Eaten plain, or mixed with plain yogurt, it can allay a craving for sweets. Also get a bag or can of shelled, unsalted nuts—pecans, walnuts or almonds are good—and, if you're planning to make granola or muffins, some raisins. The nuts will have to be refrigerated after they are opened to prevent rancidity, just like the wheat germ, the bran and the flour. The same goes for peanut butter—buy it in the supermarket only if it carries an un-hydrogenated brand. Hydrogenation, a high-heat process, counts as processing. Read the label, and if your market doesn't carry unprocessed peanut butter, get it at the health food store.

THE WEEKLY LIST

We're now getting around to the weekly shopping list—the dairy aisle, the bread, the chicken and fish, the perishable vegetables and fruit. Read all the bread labels if you're not in the habit of doing it, and pick the one that seems to offer the most whole grain per dollar. Items like caramel coloring may indicate that the bread is not really whole wheat. Rye and pumpernickel can be fine too; again, read the label. Thomas's has whole wheat English muffins now, and a lot of stores carry pita pockets, which make great sandwiches.

In the dairy aisle, take whatever milk suits your needs. With skim milk, of course, you'll get less fat, but also less vitamin A; unless the skim milk is fortified with vitamin A, it contains 0 units as compared with 1,560 per quart of whole milk. Please do not buy margarine or processed cheese; both contain hydrogenated fats, which, according to the most respected nutrition authorities, do not support health and may actually be harmful. Unless you have a cholesterol problem, butter is probably better for you than margarine. And, as Nathan Pritikin points out, margarine may not contain any cholesterol (only animal foods do), but it does contain as much fat, to say nothing of chemicals. Use butter sparingly if need be; you can make a lower-cholesterol spread by blending butter with some of the cold-pressed oil you are going to buy at the health food store, and keeping it on hand in a small tub or dish in the refrigerator. This will help cut the expense of the butter too; but remember you will also be saving money and eating less fat and much less cholesterol if you are not eating much meat. Cottage cheese can also be used in lieu of butter, hard cheese or even mayonnaise by those on restricted diets.

While in the dairy aisle, buy eggs and a large container of plain yogurt. This must be a yogurt that says "live" or "active" cultures on the label, like Dannon. If you don't like plain yogurt, buy some anyway. You can sweeten it yourself with fruit, and it is invaluable in cooking (as a sour cream or sweet cream substitute to reduce fat and calorie intake), in salad dressings, tuna salad and lots of other things. And no one will be the wiser except the cook.

Yogurt and other sour milk products—like the more liquid kefir and even cultured buttermilk—are good food for several reasons. They are high in protein, of course, being milk products. They are lower in fat than whole milk. Their lactic-acid content gives them an interestingly tangy flavor that adds sparkle to dishes, making them good substitutes for sour cream or whole milk or even mayonnaise in salads, dressings, sauces and baked goods.

They are made by use of bacterial cultures, popularly called "friendly flora" or "friendly bacteria"; in the intestinal tract, they aid in digestion and the production of B vitamins. The helpful lactobacillus acidophilus is one of the bacteria that settle in the intestines, where it aids—among other things—in the digestion of lactose, or milk sugar. This makes the fermented milk products acceptable and even desirable for some people who suffer from lactose intolerance. The lactobacillus' role in restoring B vitamins to the intestines after they have been depleted by the use of antibiotics has

DID YOU KNOW? You can make a lower-cholesterol spread by blending butter with cold-pressed oil. Keep it handy in the refrigerator.

long been an accepted fact in Europe, where doctors routinely prescribe yogurt *with* the antibiotic. Doctors in this country have begun doing so too, especially since it appears that in women, the consumption of yogurt with antibiotics can prevent yeast infections.

Only fermented milk products that contain *active* cultures can provide the lactobacillus, which is why it's important to buy cultured milk products with the cultures still alive and not pasteurized. (The sweet acidophilus milk now on the market has been scientifically developed to allow sweet milk flavor and live cultures, but most cultured milk products are sour. When pasteurized milk goes bad, it does not sour, because it is pasteurized. Raw milk, however, does sour, and it may be used like buttermilk.)

Naturally, if you cook the yogurt—in baked goods, for instance—you will destroy the lactobacillus. But you will still get the benefit of the relatively low-fat and high-protein content of the product. To take advantage of the lactobacillus, eat the yogurt uncooked in salad dressings, or add it to sauces after the heat has been turned off, stirring vigorously. This will also keep the yogurt from curdling, although if it does it will taste just as good.

CHEESES

If you're eliminating meats, dairy foods can become a real stopgap, since so many dairy dishes are already familiar—soufflés, omelets, lasagne, even a grilled cheese sandwich. It is important to get the most food value possible out of the cheese, so don't buy any cheeses that say "processed" or "cheese product" on the label. Go for the real thing. Mild Cheddar, colby, Monterey Jack, and longhorn are good all-purpose cheeses, and buying the house brand is a minor economy, although cheese prices have risen to the point where it is no longer a really cheap food. But it is a concentrated food; you might easily eat a quarter of a pound or even a half pound of meat at a meal, but you'd be unlikely to eat that much cheese. In a pinch, any mild cheese goes perfectly well even in dishes that call for the more expensive mozzarella. Cheese, like bread and butter, can be frozen for convenience.

EGGS

Of course all the eggs in the supermarkets are unfertilized, and so in a sense you might say they are "processed" too. But unless you are ready to commit yourself to the more expensive and less convenient purchase of fertilized eggs at a health food store or other source, at this point just grin and bear it. This is a gradual process, remember, and while purists may disagree, I do believe that convenience is essential to making a change in habits work.

ABOUT THOSE DRINKING HABITS

And speaking of habits, what we drink is important, too. Coffee and colas, those liquid pillars of the American way, are better used to corrode the plumbing in your house; it at least is replaceable. Both typically contain caffeine and are acidic. Soda drinks, even without caffeine or sugar, contain carbonates, and these form acids in the mouth that contribute to tooth decay. Commercial pekoe teas contain caffeine, tannic acid and dyes.

In place of sodas, try fruit juices, canned or bottled, that contain no added sugar—only what occurs in the fruit. A shot of Perrier or unsalted seltzer water can be added to fruit juice to produce a pleasing, mildly carbonated effect, at a fraction of the cost of sparkling cider, and is nice for people who want something to drink at parties besides alcohol. I find that you can bring your own apple juice and Perrier to a party and 99 percent of the people won't know or care what you're drinking.

For hot drinks, more and more markets are carrying herb teas. Brands to look for are Celestial Seasonings, Magic Mountain and some of the Bigelow and Lipton teas (but some of the latter contain caffeine—read the labels). Mint teas are an especially comforting substitute for regular tea and can be laced with milk. The flavors of camomile or rose hips put some people off at first, but both are old standbys of folk medicine and health spas, and so are fairly common ingredients. The rose hips also happen to be loaded with vitamin C. Keep trying them from time to time if you don't take to them at first. However, they don't mix well with milk.

The herb teas also provide a delightful summer alternative to sodas. Make a large batch and store it in the refrigerator in a large bottle for "instant" iced tea. If you want it sweet, add honey before it cools so the honey will dissolve.

If you are a real coffee addict, there are two or three ways to help you come down off the caffeine plateau. First is decaffeinated coffee, but commercial decaffeinated coffee is often alcohol-processed, leaving a residue that may be dangerous. Look for water-processed decaffeinated coffee, available at some health food and gourmet stores; it is usually imported from Europe and is correspondingly expensive, which is certainly an incentive to drink less of it. One Dutch brand available in some stores is Rombout's. If you find disincentives helpful, Frances Moore Lappe's Food First organization reports that coffee growers in Latin America are still using DDT on their crops, even though its use in this country has been prohibited for many years because of the damage it causes to various animals along the food chain.

There are two non-caffeinous alternatives that are worth a try. One is a carob/mint mixture called Breakaway, designed especially for coffee drinkers and sold in health food stores. The other is good old Postum, sold in grocery stores. Both have in common with coffee a slight bitterness, a faintly gritty texture and a laxative effect. Postum has malt in it, which adds sweetness. Both go well with milk.

MEANWHILE, BACK AT THE MEAT COUNTER

All you will need to buy here is chicken or other poultry. Isn't that a liberating thought? No fatty beef, no processed, salt-laden lunch meat, no cholesterol-packed bacon or lamb chops. And think of the money you'll save. Buy chicken in whatever form you like. I like whole cut-up fryers for the price, variety of pieces and convenience. Uncut chickens, of course, are usually even cheaper.

Buy fish at the supermarket unless you have a convenient local fish store. Fresh is best when it comes to fish, but frozen can do if disguised in a chowder or under some seasoning.

Commonly available fish are of several sorts. The white-fleshed fish like sole, flounder, halibut and hake are mild tasting. Cod is white and flaky but stronger and more "fishy" tasting. Tilefish, a recently popular fish, is somewhat bland. The darker fish are oilier and therefore stronger tasting. These include weakfish, bluefish, mackerel and tuna. Monk-fish, another recent marketing discovery, has been called "poor man's lobster"; it does have a firm texture, but not much flavor. Fresh salmon has a fine, mild flavor and delightfully firm texture. For non-fish lovers, sole and flounder are probably the easiest fish to like. Freshwater fish, where available, are quite tasty and generally mild, with delicate flesh. They do have a distinctly different, almost earthy flavor by comparison with saltwater fish.

ONE LAST STOP

Back to the vegetable and fruit aisle for the perishables you plan to use in the next few days—the spinach, lettuce, mushrooms, squash and bananas. You are now ready to leave the market with your month's supply of staples and a week's worth of perishables. You have completely bypassed at least one whole aisle of junk food—cookies, crackers, candies, cakes, pretzels, chips, dips, spreads and pickles, to say nothing of TV dinners, sodas, coffee and nondairy creamer. You don't need any of it. And think of the money you aren't spending on it.

Of course you stopped to buy paper towels and soap and stuff, but you're not planning to eat any of that. A last look back: the frozen food aisle. For most of what's there, fresh is better. A few exceptions: corn and peas make nice occasional additions to soup, and you can keep a package in the freezer and just use a half a handful at a time—they pop out like little marbles. Also, both vegetables are seasonal, making frozen a good alternative. For our family, frozen orange juice is in the category of emergency supplies—it's nice to have on hand for unexpected Sunday morning visitors, or whatever. And so is ice cream, for dinner guests, also unexpected. But for heaven's sake read the label. There is a difference in ingredients, even in ice cream.

STAGE ONE: MIDPOINT

By now you have stopped eating red meat and have cut down or eliminated caffeine and refined sugar from your diet. You are eating more vegetables, fruits and cereals. Your major sources of protein are chicken and other poultry, fish, milk products, eggs, lentils, peas, beans, nuts, peanut butter and whole grain products. Secondary sources are most vegetables and fruits, since they also contain some protein.

You are also incorporating certain foods into your diet regularly to get your share of some important vitamins and minerals:

Vitamin A: eggs, yellow fruits and vegetables (citrus fruits, apricots, cantaloupe, squashes, carrots), green leafy vegetables, milk products

B vitamins: poultry, fish, whole grains, legumes, nuts, eggs, milk products, green leafy vegetables

Vitamin C: citrus fruits, tomatoes and peppers, cantaloupe, strawberries, alfalfa sprouts, rose hips, the cabbage family

Vitamin D: fortified milk and milk products, eggs

Vitamin E: cold-pressed oils, eggs, wheat germ, sweet potatoes

Calcium: milk products, green leafy vegetables, shellfish

Potassium: vegetables, fruits, whole grains, legumes

Iron: poultry, fish, eggs, green leafy vegetables, dried fruits

Magnesium: seafood, whole grains, dark green vegetables, nuts

GOOD NEWS:

 A typical day of Stage One menus gives you 1½ times the adult RDA of protein. (For example, you might eat half a cup of cereal for breakfast, with 4 ounces of milk and 4 ounces yogurt; a cup of lentil soup for lunch; steamed fish and rice for dinner.)

 Your day's menus give you the required RDA of vitamin A and the B vitamins and twice the required amount of vitamin C. (For example, for breakfast you might have a glass of orange juice and a banana; your lunch includes a salad of lettuce, cabbage, carrots and green peppers in a pita pocket, plus an apple; at dinner you have a baked sweet potato or broccoli and a salad of lettuce and escarole.) You get your RDA of vitamin E and some additional vitamin C with a salad dressing of cold-pressed oil and lemon juice.

✔ Your sodium intake from three meals, excluding table salt, is less than one-tenth the average daily intake for adult Americans. You can add one teaspoon of salt to the day's meals and still be at the low end of the average daily intake. Your potassium intake is well within the average daily intake, thanks to the lentil soup, fruits and vegetables.

FOUR

WHO NEEDS A BANQUET?

Stage One meals are designed with the whole family in mind, meat eaters too. With the basic supplies in your kitchen you'll never be without a good dozen options for a dinner that can be cooked in about an hour, with a minimum of fuss and without any advance planning on your part. I'm not saying it will be a banquet—and who needs one?—but it certainly won't be junk food either. What it might be is: rice and vegetables; one of several hearty homemade soups, including minestrone, potage à la bonne femme, pea or lentil, with or without a toasted cheese sandwich on the side; an omelet, quiche or vegetable pie; or a pasta dish, from tuna noodle casserole to linguine with clam sauce. And that's just with the basics, the supplies that keep for weeks at a time.

At our house, these dinners evolved as an answer to what two working people—the beleaguered vegetarian chef and her sympathetic meat-eating spouse—were going to eat at 8 o'clock on a weekday night.

By adding more perishable items here or there, I found I could make more exotic but equally easy dishes, from spinach vichyssoise to pasta primavera. All in an hour or less, with minimal advance planning. The trick with the perishables was to be sure to use them the week they were purchased.

I also found that on nights when the meat eater absolutely craved a hamburger or steak, dual menus could be arranged, featuring meat for Paul and something vegetable for me. It wasn't too much trouble because most nights we ate the same foods. Thinking ahead also made it easier, cooking large batches of things to last for several days—soups, meatless lasagne, stewed chicken, a turkey that would eventually become soup with homemade noodles. Lasagne, soups, homemade marinara sauce—these could all be frozen too, in large batches or individual portions for later use.

One thing I found when I was first starting to expand my repertoire of vegetable dishes was that I was handicapped by a lifetime of eating frozen or canned vegetables. I didn't know how to clean spinach or mushrooms, or dismember broccoli; and many varieties of vegetables, from kale to rutabagas, were just unknown.

Now I find that I have to curb my enthusiasm in the vegetable aisle. The thing is, unless you are planning to feed a multitude, or are a real vegetable lover, you'll find that if you buy some of everything that looks good, a lot of stuff will get wasted. I for one don't have the energy to work a full-time job and also experiment with new recipes every night. With that in mind, I usually buy no more than two perishable vegetables at a time, or three or four if I'm planning on a lot of salad. When they are used up, I buy something else, relying on the tougher staple vegetables in between.

Herewith a checklist of the vegetables commonly found in markets, some of them probably dearer to your heart than others, all with possibilities for the vegetarian menu.

THE COLE FAMILY

Members of this group include cabbage, kale, collards, cauli-flower, brussels sprouts, kohlrabi and broccoli. They are rich in vitamin C, comparing favorably with citrus fruit; the darker green members, like brussels sprouts, kale and broc-coli, have lots of vitamin A. These are strongly flavored vege-tables, and the secret is not to cook them to death. Boiled in traditional fashion, they are soggy and disagreeable. They should be steamed or sautéed until they are barely done. The flavor of the cabbage, especially, profits from sautéing. Be-cause of their sturdiness, they are valuable as ingredients in vegetarian entrées. Broccoli is a good addition to stir-fry or pasta. Mustard greens and turnips are genetically members of this group and are covered in categories that follow.

LEAFY GREENS

Lettuce, escarole, endives, spinach, Swiss chard and water-cress are available in supermarkets. Other greens include mustard greens, dandelion, and the leaves of beets, turnips and other vegetables. These are rich in vitamin A and chloro-phyll—the greener the plant, the more chlorophyll; and the more chlorophyll, the more iron. Iron in turn helps build healthy hemoglobin, increasing the oxygen-carrying capacity of the blood. In an environment laden with toxins, the greens are especially valuable. It is virtually impossible to eat too much of them. If they are eaten raw, it is difficult to consume much volume because of their bulk. When cooked by steam-ing or sautéing, however, they wilt to a fraction of their raw size. The darker greens have a bitter taste that is modified by cooking them in the traditional Italian way, sautéing them with a little garlic and covering them to steam for a minute. Soy sauce can be added in lieu of salt before covering. The lighter greens, of course, are salad favorites. Try mixing the milder, blander greens with darker, more bitter greens in salad for added flavor and food value. Don't buy more than a couple of kinds at a time—they wilt quickly.

THE SQUASHES

Certain summer and winter squashes are commonly found in groceries. The soft-skinned summer squashes include the yellow, the white patty pan and the zucchini. These are endlessly useful as they are plentiful in summer, lending their delicate meat to dishes ranging from stir-fry to ratatouille to lasagne. Their texture, flavor and bulk make them admirable as the centerpiece of a meal; they must not be overcooked or they become mushy and watery. The winter squashes, including the acorn, Hubbard, butternut and turban, have a rather sweet, starchy flesh, like that of yams but with more texture and taste. They are a good side dish or ingredient for grain dishes. They can be used like their relative the pumpkin in pie or breads.

A recent novelty in the supermarket is the spaghetti squash, whose flesh when baked or parboiled shreds into spaghetti-like strands, a fine substitute for people who are unable to eat wheat products or are simply looking for variety.

ROOTS

Carrots are a mainstay of a vegetarian diet. They are cheap, keep well, are rich in vitamin A, and can be used in virtually any dish from stew to cake. Less familiar in this country are turnips, parsnips and rutabagas. A good way to start into a vegetarian diet—or simply stretch a meat diet, as centuries of cooks have done—is to include these roots in stews, thus augmenting the quantity and quality of the vegetable portion of the meal. Rutabagas are an especially sweet and tasty vegetable in stew or casseroles; parsnips are like a sweeter carrot, and often are a good bargain in winter.

The onion is another mainstay, whose presence is indispensable in all entrées. Cooking takes the bite out of it, making it a sweet vegetable. In the onion family are scallions, shallots, garlic and leeks, all of which are rendered mild by steaming, which expresses the volatile oils that give them their characteristic strong flavor. Beets are earthly no matter how you slice them, but rich in iron and highly recommended as food for the blood. For starters, eating them with acid foods helps offset their "beety" flavor, which is why pickled beets and borscht, containing vinegar, are palatable even to confirmed beet-haters.

THE NIGHTSHADE FAMILY

What would we do without these once exotic fruits that caused such alarm when first introduced into Europe? Members of this family include the tomato and the potato, eggplant and peppers. They are excluded from a strict macrobiotic diet by some, or used sparingly, but they are all absolutely invaluable in making the transition from a meat diet, for the flavor and variety they provide. The tomatoes and peppers are an excellent source of vitamin C, and the potatoes of potassium, some protein and even vitamin C. The eggplant is especially valuable as a meat alternative because it works well as an entrée. It also allays a craving for meat.

BEANS AND PEAS

Cooked green or snap beans make a good side dish or ingredient in stir-fry, or can be eaten cold in salads. They should not be boiled for 20 minutes in a quart of water, as some standard recipes suggest, but steamed or cooked in a scant amount of water until barely tender. Broad beans, like limas, are not often found in supermarkets. They must be hulled and can be steamed or boiled lightly. What are found in supermarkets increasingly are snow peas, those glamorous participants in many an Oriental dish. Very delicate, they need minimal cooking. Dried legumes, of course, are central to vegetarian fare, because of their high protein content and satisfying taste and texture.

AMONG OTHERS

Celery, actually considered an herb, is as universal in dishes as carrots and onions. So are mushrooms, which, like squash and eggplant, can replace meat as a central flavor and texture. Parsley and watercress are both rich in chlorophyll, texture and flavor. Cucumbers, a relative of the melons, are too delicate for cooking but excellent in cold soups and salads. Bean sprouts, bought at market or started at home, are rich in protein and add texture and flavor to salads and main dishes. Avocados, asparagus and artichokes are delicacies gobbled up by their fans in season. Asparagus is a good source of vitamin A, and the fatty avocado contains vitamin E. Artichokes aren't rich in much of anything except possibly fun.

FRUITS

Fresh fruits, except apples and citrus fruits, are too perishable to be called staples. But they're great weapons in combating the sugar habit, and when eaten plain, in cleansing and nourishing the body. Pritikin recommends them to his patients as a major element of their low-fat diet, suggesting up to five pieces of fruit daily, with juice to substitute for no more than one of these. How many of us can claim to eat even one piece of fruit a day, if juice is excepted?

Good places to sandwich them into a day are at breakfast (yes, you do have time to section a grapefruit), for desserts, and in lieu of the deadly coffee break. Peeling an orange is a good way around the caffeine temptation—the aroma of citrus is guaranteed to distract your olfactory nerve until the danger is past, and you can still be companionable. If sticky fingers offend you, carry a cleansing towelette in your lunch box, briefcase or whatever.

Why such detail over a bunch of bananas and such? Because the habits they can replace in most of us are such bad ones, and so ingrained, that our devious subconscious will present endless justifications for not changing our ways: It's too much trouble; peaches are messy; where will I spit the seeds; I can't get through the afternoon without coffee, I'll fall asleep; what would the boss think if he saw orange peels all over my desk; I'll ruin my clean shirt; you've got to be kidding, me sit here in front of everybody and eat a banana with the skin dangling down all over the place?

It's good to get attuned to when fruits are in and out of season—citrus fruits are a welcome bargain at winter's end, when nothing else is in season, but at summer's end, when everything else is ripe and cheap, the lemons and oranges are tired-looking and expensive. Summer fruits start with strawberries, run through peaches, blueberries, plums and melons, and end with the pears and apples of fall. The fruits are, of course, best and cheapest at the height of their season, and you can freeze a hoard of your favorites to cheer you up periodically throughout the winter.

FIVE

BACK TO THE HEALTH FOOD STORE

For the time being, trips to the health food store can be quick and infrequent—and inexpensive. You need your health food store if your grocery store can't provide: cold-pressed oil; sea salt; tamari or lima soy sauce; raw honey. Optional: unhydrogenated peanut butter; herbal teas; carob powder as a chocolate substitute.

The reason you need cold-pressed oil, usually available only in health food stores, is that commercially available oils are prepared either under intense heat and pressure or by the solvent method of extraction, in which a chemical solvent —usually petroleum based—extracts the oil from its source. Traces of the solvent may remain in the oil. Refined oil is further heated and treated with bleach for cosmetic purposes.

Commercial oils may also be hydrogenated, that is, subjected to a high-heat process in which additional hydrogen atoms are added to the individual molecules. If hydrogenated, oils cannot become rancid, which is why the process is frequently used on the fats that will go onto supermarket shelves in bottles, jars of peanut butter, or cakes, cookies and crackers. Hydrogenation provides a form of stability in the attachment of hydrogen atoms to the molecular chain that is a fat, or lipid.

Rancidity occurs when the molecular chain acquires extra oxygen atoms. The fat is then prematurely oxidized; oxidation would normally occur during digestion. The reason both rancid and hydrogenated fats are to be avoided is that both represent a fat that is saturated.

The price we pay for ingesting saturated fats, fats that cannot be effectively digested and used by the body, is that we carry them as an added burden in the bloodstream, where they clog arteries and cause atherosclerosis, and in our overworked tissues, which become starved for oxygen. By impeding the metabolism of food and the removal of wastes in the body, the fats also contribute to gout and diabetes. Almost half the caloric intake of Americans today is in fats, many of them saturated.

The fats most easily digested are the unsaturated fats found in cold-pressed oils. Good oils to buy are sesame (lightweight Hain brand or medium-weight Eden brand) for general cooking and for salads, or olive oil for Mediterranean dishes. (Olive oil, however, is fairly heavy and should not be used for general cooking.) These are the two oils most likely to be genuinely cold pressed because that is the method that works best on olives and sesame seeds. Other oils labeled "cold processed" may be cold pressed, or may have been processed at a low level of heat. If sesame oil is not available,

---

DID YOU KNOW? Cold-pressed oils are preferable to commercially prepared oils, which are often extracted from the seed by use of a chemical solvent, traces of which may remain in the oil. Refined oils are also treated with bleach for cosmetic purposes.

---

safflower and corn oil are probably the best substitutes. Corn and safflower also are good oils for baked goods.

SWEETENERS

Raw honey is a more natural product than processed commercial sugars, but it is still a form of sugar and as such is an extreme food, not meant to be eaten in quantity. It consists mostly of simple sugars (monosaccharides), and contains traces of vitamins, minerals and antibiotics. It will not spoil, but may crystallize in time. It can be liquefied by setting it in warm water; or the crystallized honey can be used in place of sugar in recipes. Do *not* believe any recipe that tells you to substitute honey for sugar on a unit-for-unit basis. Honey is several times sweeter than sugar and should be used sparingly.

Do not feed honey to infants under the age of one; their systems cannot digest it, and infant botulism may result.

Blackstrap molasses may also be used sparingly as a sugar substitute; it contains iron and B vitamins. Be sure to get the unsulfured kind. Used in conjunction with honey, it is an excellent brown sugar substitute. Use just a little at first until you get used to the taste; then use more blackstrap in proportion to the honey for a richer taste.

Try cutting the amount of sweetener called for in recipes by one-third or even one-half. Remember, the recipe wasn't tailored to your needs. If a recipe calls for two tablespoons of sugar, try using half a tablespoon of honey, plus a teaspoon of blackstrap if brown sugar is indicated. You may have to add more liquid ingredients to compensate for the sugar.

Honey works fine in pies, puddings, fruit desserts and cookies. For cakes and breads, it may prevent them from rising properly because it is heavier than sugar. Experiment. Corn syrup counts as sugar, by the way, and is often used in prepared foods. Read the label!

SALT

Sea salt contains a greater variety of minerals than commercially prepared table salt, but tamari—the common name for fermented soy, soya or shoyu sauce—is even easier for the body to handle. If you are buying sea salt, you may want to buy iodized sea salt for the time being. Later, seaweeds provide a source of iodine if you decide to use them regularly.

Tamari, says Naboru Muramoto in *Healing Ourselves*, contains 18 percent salt, compared with 2.8 percent salt in sea water, which our blood closely resembles. Table salt, in contrast, is close to 100 percent in concentration. "Salt," says Muramoto, "does not enter the cells alone, but oil and salt are held in the cell when they are combined. That is why soya sauce is good; the fat from the soybeans combines with the salt." Commercial soy sauces are not naturally fermented and often contain alcohol. Read the label, and if your soy sauce was not made by natural fermentation, go to the health food store.

WHAT ELSE?

It is also worth noting what other items your health food store stocks. Even in the realm of health foods, all stores are not equal. Some are healthier than others. Things to look for include soy products—flour and grits; miso soy paste; tofu bean curd cakes; or tempeh, an Indonesian fermented soy food. You may also want to check out the store's stock of whole wheat noodle products, cereals (looking for ones that don't contain sugar), dairy products (comparing prices with the supermarket), and the supply of grains and legumes, such as rice, buckwheat, millet, beans, peas and lentils. How are they stored—loose, or in airtight packages? If they are loose, you will want to watch the store over a period of time to see whether a high turnover guarantees freshness.

If you didn't find any herb teas in the supermarket, this is the place to buy them. If you want to eat granola and don't want to bother making it, read the labels here for one that doesn't contain any sugar, not even brown sugar.

SIX

IMPLEMENTING A STRATEGY: WHAT TO DO WITH IT ALL

So now you're back at the kitchen counter with several bags of groceries. Start by storing them properly.

■ Grains. All grain products should either be refrigerated (flour) or stored in airtight containers (whole grains). For the latter, wide-mouthed jars, such as peanut butter or Mason jars, are ideal, but juice bottles will do and in a pinch coffee cans can be used with their plastic lids or with a piece of wax paper and a rubber band for a top.

Jars with lids are preferable because moth larvae and other critters that like grain can eat through plastic wrap, paper and cardboard, or infiltrate via a lid that doesn't fit securely. If you're using a narrow-mouthed jar, save spills and aggravation by using a makeshift funnel. Just roll up a piece of clean paper into a funnel shape—wide mouth and narrow bottom—and gently pour your rice, granola or beans into the jar.

It's not a bad idea to store flour in the refrigerator in canisters or plastic bags to keep it dry and free of smells, and to prevent spills. Clear storage containers make it easier to identify contents, but tins will do as long as you label them. Nail polish is good for this, as well as for labeling freezer-bound containers.

■ Oils. Store in the refrigerator when not in use.

■ Sweeteners. Raw honey may be stored on the shelf. Don't worry if it crystallizes. It can be liquefied easily by heating. Just set the bottle in a pan of water over a low flame. Or use crystallized honey in baking. Maple syrup molds unless stored in the refrigerator.

■ Nuts. In their shells, nuts may be stored in any cool, dry place for months. But shelled or broken nut meats keep better if refrigerated. Unhydrogenated peanut butter does better in the refrigerator if you are keeping it more than a week.

■ Large quantities. Bread, butter and cheese can all be frozen if you've found a bargain or don't want to get caught short. Butter and cheese periodically go on sale, and even if it's only once or twice a year, it's worth stocking up if you have room.

BASIC TOOLS

The foods you're fixing will be steamed, boiled, sautéed, baked and occasionally broiled, or they'll be eaten raw in salads or as finger food. There is nothing particularly mysterious about cooking vegetarian foods, or about the tools to do it with. It helps to have good-quality kitchen equipment no matter what you're cooking. It can make the difference between enjoyment and a hassle. But the equipment can be pretty basic.

You'll want a large pot to cook soups and boil pasta; a smaller pot with a tight-fitting lid for boiling rice; a large skillet or wok for sautéing and stir-frying vegetables; a small skillet; a pie pan and one or two casserole dishes or pans for

DID YOU KNOW? Aluminum leaching from pots into the cooking water adds aluminum salts to the food, which can upset your body's mineral balance. Stainless steel should not be scoured heavily, according to studies that showed scouring could release toxic amounts of nickel and chromium.

the oven; a scrub brush; a colander; a spatula; a ladle; a sieve or skimmer; a grater; a couple of wooden spoons; a good sharp small knife and cutting board; mixing bowls; and a rotary beater. A blender or food processor is handy but not necessary. Things like quiche pans and cleavers are refinements, and fine if you have them, but also not necessary. A big bread board and a couple of muffin tins are a nice addition if you plan to try baking. An inexpensive plastic rotary salad spinner can save a lot of work drying leafy greens.

Do not use aluminum pots for boiling or steaming vegetables; the aluminum leaches into the cooking water and adds aluminum salts to the food, and this can upset your body's mineral balance. Probably the best cookware is enameled iron ware, but it is expensive. Stainless steel is all right if it is not scoured heavily, which, according to some studies, can release toxic nickel and chromium. If using a thin enameled pot, get a flamespreader from the hardware store to prevent excess heat from causing foods to stick. Iron skillets are fine. For baking, glass ovenproof dishes are best, but in a pinch even the foil type from the grocery store will do. You can steam foods in a stainless steel colander, but a stainless steel steamer—available in hardware stores, grocery stores and health food shops—is much handier and a good $3 investment.

PREPARATION TECHNIQUES

Washing and cutting up vegetables is probably the most tedious part of vegetarian cooking. It is essential to find a system that works for you, or you will be driven to convenience foods in short order.

One thing that helps is that you can stop peeling your root vegetables (carrots and potatoes), unless they have really tough hides (onions, some turnips). Likewise the squashes, eggplants and apples. Just scrub them thoroughly under running water or in a bowl of water, and set them aside to drain.

The leafy vegetables are among the most cumbersome to wash and drain. A good method is to keep a dishpan just for washing vegetables. When washing loose-leaf lettuce, spinach, escarole and the like, draw a panful of cold water, add the leaves, swish them around, trim if necessary (by pulling off spinach stems, for instance) and set to drain in the colander, lined with a clean dish towel. If you don't have a salad spinner, you can speed up drying by the time-honored expedient of wrapping the leaves securely in the towel and whirling it rapidly at arm's length so that excess water flies outward. This will spray the surrounding area, so do it outside or in a spot you don't mind getting wet.

With carrots and summer squash, you need only trim the ends, and that's mostly for aesthetics. With potatoes, cut out any eyes or spoiled spots; for eggplants the stem end; with peppers the stem and core. Mushrooms should be cleaned by wiping with a damp towel; don't wash them or they'll get soggy. Cabbage can be rinsed and dried before storing in the refrigerator; then just slice off thin cross-sections as needed. If the cabbage blackens along the cut edge, just slice this portion off before cutting what you'll use. To prepare broccoli for cooking, chop off the tough end of the stem, rinse and split into quarters or even smaller sections; cook and eat the little leaves, or freeze them for soup. Broccoli stems also can be peeled and cooked by themselves if you want to use the florets separately. Brussels sprouts are cleaned by cutting off the stem tip and cross-hatching the stem end with a knife. Cauliflower is cleaned like broccoli.

Cooks often refer to two aesthetically pleasing types of slices for vegetables: julienne and nituke. They are both basically rectangular and give your dishes a more pleasing appearance and texture. And because they are thinly cut, they cook quickly. You're doubtless acquainted with julienned slices from chef salads, where the ham and cheese are julienned; the nituke slices are often described as match-stick, as seen in some nouvelle cuisine dishes, most often for carrots or zucchini. I find the easiest way to nituke carrots and zucchini is to cut round slices first, then stack them and slice into match-sticks. Carrots may also be sliced in rounds across the grain; the trick here is to slice diagonally in very thin slices, so the rounds are really exaggerated ovals. Mushrooms are best cut in thin cross-sections of cap and stem; peppers can be cut in strips and then chopped; onions can conveniently be chopped after peeling by cross-hatching the surface of one sliced end, then slicing through the onion as if to make rounds.

COOKING BEANS AND RICE

Most grains and legumes come with cooking instructions, but several things are worth noting.

■ Dried beans are best soaked overnight before cooking and then baked or simmered for a couple of hours. But there is a shortcut. Rinse the beans, discard any that are badly shriveled, and bring to a boil in twice the amount of water needed to cover. Boil for 2 minutes and remove from heat. Let stand for 1 hour, tightly covered. Then cook for 2 hours, or until done.

■ While cooking dried beans is going to take at least a couple of hours, even if you take shortcuts, split peas and lentils both go fairly fast—much faster than most directions say, in fact—and often are done in half an hour to an hour.

■ Brown rice will absorb two to three times its own volume of liquid in cooking—so 1 cup of rice cooks in 2 or 3 cups of water. The rice should be rinsed, then put in the pan with cold water and a little salt, and brought to a boil. If necessary, skim any scum off the surface, then cover with a tight-fitting lid and turn down the heat. After a few minutes, check to make sure the water is boiling; otherwise your heat is too low. Then cover and leave it for half an hour. Check at a half hour only to see if all the water is gone, and if the rice is about done (eat a grain). If the rice is still hard and you need to add water, add just a little—a quarter cup or less—and re-cover. If the water is all gone —you can tell by listening for the sound of boiling—and the rice is nearly done, simply re-cover and turn off the heat. It will steam itself done. On no account should you stir the rice before you're ready to eat it; this will make it gummy. If you don't get perfect rice the first time, do not panic and conclude that you can't cook rice. Basically only two things can go wrong with rice: too much liquid will make it soggy; too little and the rice will not be cooked or

---

DID YOU KNOW? If you don't get perfect brown rice the first time, don't panic. Really only two things can go wrong with rice: too much liquid or not enough. Your nose will alert you before any more than the bottom of the pot is burned—eat the rest of the rice and soak the pot overnight.

---

will burn. However, your nose will alert you before any
more than the bottom is burned; and the rest will be fine.
And remember what Michel Abehsera says in his *Zen
Macrobiotic Cooking* (Avon Books; 1968): Burned rice is
good for you. Your body likes the carbon. As for the pot,
soak it overnight with baking soda.

FOR STARTERS, DINNER

With the information and supplies you have on hand, you can
easily make a dinner of stir-fried vegetables over rice; a pot of
chicken stew; a simple meal of steamed vegetables; or a more
elaborate repast of vegetables over pasta with a light cheese
sauce.

But first, a thought about menu planning. The way it is
usually presented, you'd think they were mass-producing the
meals somewhere up in Consumer Heaven. The plans seem
to assume that every day of the week you are going to have
the same components in your meal—an entrée, two vegetables, salad or salad substitute, bread, butter, dessert and a
beverage. So these menu plans are virtually useless for anyone whose life lacks a cookie-cutter regularity, or who simply
doesn't want to eat a huge meal—the same huge meal, basically—seven nights a week.

These so-called menus also presume that you're never going to have any leftovers, or eat the same thing two nights in a
row, or make up a big batch of something to eat all week.

Needless to say, this is not my idea of sane menu planning.
What works best for the busy person is perhaps a modicum of
variety in ingredients coupled with simplicity in preparation.

The recipes for Stage One are based on that assumption.
They offer you a couple of weeks' worth of recipes for main
dishes that will provide adequate nutritional elements if
eaten as a meal in themselves, or that can be augmented with

side dishes if you are especially hungry or are entertaining. All these main dishes can be put together in about an hour, sometimes less. Many of them require nothing more than the staples you bought in Chapter 3. If you're ready to start cooking, just move right to the recipes and come back for breakfast and lunch later.

BREAKFAST AND LUNCH

For breakfast, since most people are just trying to get on with the day at this point, what's simplest is probably best. Please eat some fruit for breakfast instead of starting your day with a jolt of coffee. There's no rule that says you can't have fruit juice and more fruit as well; the sugars in the fruit will help you wake up if you're missing your coffee.

Cereal leaves you with the option of eating eggs at another meal, but you could also go the route of toast fortified with cottage cheese or peanut butter. If you're not hungry when you first get up, pack half a sandwich or some fruit or yogurt for a mid-morning snack.

For winter mornings, there's nothing wrong with your favorite hot cereal five days a week and something fancier on weekends. Try cooking oatmeal and pouring cooked apples— just slice and cook in a little water with cinnamon or nutmeg —over it. Add milk or yogurt if desired, and maple sugar or honey occasionally for variety. If you like prunes, cooked pitted prunes are also good over hot cereal, as are raisins and nuts. One way or another, you can give yourself all the variety you need, plus a nice feeling of warmth to start the day.

I like to top cold cereal with a mixture of half milk and half plain yogurt shaken in a jar—a frothy, smooth and delicious topping.

For lunch, the possibilities depend on whether you eat out a lot, have access to a company cafeteria, or pack lunch. Once again, you must know yourself; there's no point getting frustrated and out of sorts by trying to pack your lunch if you've always eaten out. Better to try to find a place where you can eat out at least some of the time and not have to eat a really heavy or processed meal. But if you pack your lunch, and have always done so, you can coordinate your lunches with your meals at home. Or you can try a combination of both strategies.

If you're packing lunch, some relatively quick and easy possibilities are:

- Soup from whatever's in the pot this week, packed in a wide-mouthed Thermos.
- A peanut butter and sliced apple sandwich.
- A cheese sandwich on whole wheat bread, with lettuce, tomato and sprouts.
- Salad packed in a container with a small bottle of home-made dressing on the side.
- A salad stuffed into a pita pocket, with dressing, cottage cheese or tuna to be added later, packed separately.

Only you know how much you will want to eat before you get home again. Take enough food so that you won't turn to junk food in desperation. This could mean an extra sandwich, a Thermos of something hot every day, supplemental pieces of fruit or containers of yogurt or other snacks. Try, however, to avoid eating so much that you feel logy and overfed, since this will only drive you to want coffee or sweets to jolt you awake.

Two suggestions for salad eaters. If you know you are going to pack a salad every day, you should make up salad dressing in large batches. And you may also want to clean and shred several days' worth of vegetables at a time—lettuce, cabbage, carrots and peppers. Things like tomatoes, cucumbers, bean sprouts, onions and avocados can be added daily, if you want them. This cuts down on preparation time when you're in a hurry, and the salad mix can be stored in an airtight plastic container in the refrigerator until needed. Vegetables lose nutrients, of course, when they're cut up, but what we're seeking for starters is a workable balance of nutrition and convenience.

DINING OUT

Since the advent of nouvelle cuisine cooking and a general consciousness-raising in the field of health, restaurants almost invariably offer something good in the way of seafood, quiche, or vegetable dishes. Even places that used to emphasize beef have put fish on the menu, and usually offer a salad bar. But in places where beef is the forte, you may find the aromas too distracting to make anything else a treat. That's why it is helpful to go someplace completely new and different while breaking old habits. There may even be a vegetarian restaurant within reach, and any good Italian or Chinese restaurant will have nonmeat dishes. Japanese restaurants concentrate heavily on fish and vegetables, often cooking them at your table. Even diners offer eggs and fish, though they may lean heavily on fried food, and that's not really good.

The thornier problem by far is eating at someone's house. If in doubt, you can tell the host that you're not eating much meat these days. Close friends may already have figured this out, and planned something everyone will enjoy. If not, they certainly won't be offended, and you can always offer to bring something of your own.

As for eating meat once in a while, it depends on why you have become a vegetarian. If you are convinced that killing animals is wrong, then of course you cannot eat the meat. It will probably help everyone if you say so simply and don't argue about it, especially over dinner. If you are becoming a vegetarian for reasons of personal spiritual enlightenment, you may find the idea of the setback from eating meat too depressing to be worthwhile, and will act accordingly.

If, however, you are somewhere in the great middle ground of wishing to improve your health and provide for the world's hungry, it seems unlikely that an occasional exception will do much harm, as long as it does not become an excuse for frequent exceptions and resultant disorganized eating. Because, whatever your dietary pattern, it *is* a pattern. Eating for most of us is not haphazard. And to change the pattern requires a new pattern, one that should not be undermined for frivolous reasons.

Too, your body makes whatever adjustments it must to your eating and drinking habits, be they good or bad. As you learn to eat more prudently and lightly, your body shifts gears accordingly, and you do it no favor by throwing it into reverse.

WHAT ABOUT THE FAMILY?

For adults in the family who don't choose to be vegetarian, Stage One shouldn't be much of a problem. You don't have to make a point of telling people where you put the yogurt or the tamari unless they want to know. And for children, too, the meals the family eats at home together won't have changed that much in Stage One.

If you are embarking on a vegetarian diet for specific reasons, especially moral or philosophical, the best thing to do is explain them, without proselytizing. One experienced vegetarian mother suggests that children are at least as likely as adults to understand a desire to avoid eating animals, or to help feed the hungry children of the world. The idea of health, to those who are young and have known little else, is likely to be more abstract.

But I believe allowances should be made for peer pressure, too, and that it should be clear to your children that you make these allowances. They should not be made to feel guilty about eating food in other people's houses or on a school field trip where the choice of food is not theirs—or yours.

One vegetarian mother recalls how her daughter, now 17, was excluded from a birthday party after the family decided to forgo meat six years ago. The child was told it was because "we're having hamburgers and hot dogs and you don't eat them." Everyone else in the class was invited and, says her mother, she talked about it for a long time. Since then, says the mother, non-vegetarians have become more accepting, and at a recent band picnic a younger daughter grilled tofu-based hot dogs alongside everyone else's.

The hardest thing for the children in the beginning, one family found, was not peer pressure, but passing up the fast-food hamburgers they had enjoyed. The key to their success as a vegetarian family, the mother thinks, is that she and her husband presented the idea to their children and made them part of the decision-making process. The fact that it was their own decision to be vegetarians made it possible for the children to withstand peer pressure and their own temptations.

GETTING ON WITH IT

At this point, it's time to start practicing whatever plan you have established for Stage One—shopping, cooking and enjoying. Some Stage One recipes will be good for Stage Two, and even Stage Three. Stage One recipes are chosen because of their ingredients (chicken and fish) or because their simplicity and tastiness make them an easy place to start. Take a moment to look at the recipe section and try picturing a typical week in your life incorporating some new dishes. Then, if you want, you can look ahead to Stage Two.

TWO DIETS

Compare a day of Stage One with what might have preceded it. A typical Stage One day might include:

Breakfast: 1 cup shredded wheat and granola; 1 banana; 4 ounces grapefruit juice; 4 ounces milk and 4 ounces yogurt, blended for cereal; decaffeinated coffee or Postum.

Lunch: 1 cup barley-mushroom soup; pita pocket stuffed with ¼ cup shredded cheese, lettuce, shredded cabbage and carrot, green pepper and cherry tomatoes, and dressed with a vinaigrette of lemon juice and oil; a pear.

Dinner: roast chicken, rice, a sweet potato or broccoli, a salad of lettuce and escarole, vinaigrette dressing, a glass of wine.

Your pre–Stage One day might have included:

Breakfast: orange juice, pastry, coffee.

Lunch: canned chicken soup; ham and cheese on rye.

Dinner: steak, baked potato with sour cream, salad with commercial dressing, apple pie.

GOOD NEWS:

✓ The Stage One diet offers 20 more protein grams than the pre–Stage One; 100 more carbohydrate grams; five times the fiber grams; one-seventh of the fat; and one-ninth of the sodium. The Stage One menus also provide 20 grams more protein than the RDA of 56 grams for adult American men.

THE
GRADUAL
VEGETARIAN

STAGE TWO

SEVEN

INGREDIENTS FOR HEALTH

The menus we were preparing in Stage One didn't represent a great departure from mainstream cooking. But what about *real* vegetarians, the ones who don't eat any meat?

Stage Two moves into the great middle ground of vegetarianism—with dairy foods, grains, nuts, beans and peas as the sources of protein. Since many people who consider themselves vegetarians do eat fish, we will include one or two fish recipes for festive occasions. We will also begin to look at some of the foods that are less familiar to our Western lifestyle, notably the protein-rich soy products.

And we will hope to find a positive answer to the two questions most people ask themselves about this kind of a diet: Will it keep me healthy, and will I like the way it tastes?

If the prospect of the unfamiliar seems intimidating, don't be put off. Your diet is not going to change radically unless you want it to.

First, in moving away from a traditional American diet, there is the question of whether any other diet can really provide all the nutrients you need on a long-term basis. It is only fair to say that no one really knows. Nutrition as a subject of scientific study is very young, and much of the research that has been done has been funded by sources with specific goals—proving that a lack of a certain vitamin produces a certain health problem, for example. These studies, while valuable, do not provide a total picture of what constitutes healthy nutrition. Furthermore, most of them have focused on common Western foods. There is much less research available on the nutritive value of soy foods, like miso, tofu and tempeh, or of the seaweeds. These foods are simply not in the mainstream of Western eating.

On the other hand, we are becoming more and more aware that some of the mainstream foods we have taken for granted, especially those high in fats and cholesterol, are not necessarily pillars of good nutrition. And some studies have been funded with even more specific goals in mind—such as a major industry trying to prove that its product is vital to, or not destructive of, human health. William Dufty in *Sugar Blues* (Chilton Book Co.; 1975) cites an instance of dental studies being funded by the Sugar Research Foundation. And even when research is done with no ulterior motive, human beings can be notoriously unreliable when it comes to food, and this is an obstacle to researchers.

PROTEIN: THE GREAT DEBATE

Americans have been obsessed for decades with a diet that is adequate in protein, in spite of the fact that we lead the world in protein consumption. In countries where people eat much less protein, the population as a whole does survive, much of it in health as good as our own, but our nervousness over getting that protein continues.

The meat and dairy industries profit from our further obsession with getting "complete" protein. Frances Moore Lappe's original *Diet for a Small Planet* was written in answer to that obsession. She outlined the concept of protein com-

---

DID YOU KNOW? At the center of the great protein debate are the amino acids. Of the twenty-two acids that are vital to the body's growth, tissue repair and metabolism, thirteen can be manufactured by the body itself. The other nine, which can be obtained only from food, are called "essential" for that reason.

---

plementarity in detail, showing how "incomplete" plant and grain proteins could be combined, and further enriched with dairy foods, to provide a "whole" protein adequate to human daily needs. In the new edition of her book, however, published by Ballantine in 1983, Lappe remarks that she may have gone a bit overboard:

> In 1971 I stressed protein complementarity because I assumed that the only way to get enough protein (without consuming too many calories) was to create a protein as usable by the body as animal protein. In combating the myth that meat is the only way to get high-quality protein, I reinforced another myth. I gave the impression that in order to get enough protein without meat, considerable care was needed in choosing foods. Actually, it is much easier than I thought.
>
> With three important exceptions, there is little danger of protein deficiency in a plant food diet. The exceptions are diets very heavily dependent on fruit or on some tubers, such as sweet potatoes or cassava, or on junk food (refined flours, sugars, and fat). . . . *In all other diets, if people are getting enough calories, they are virtually certain of getting enough protein.*

At the center of the great protein debate are the amino acids. Of the twenty-two amino acids that are vital to the body's growth, tissue repair and metabolism of food, thirteen can be manufactured by the body itself. The other nine, which can be obtained only from food, are called the "essential" amino acids for that reason. All the shuffling about of foods that do not contain all nine "essential" amino acids is designed to get them into our bodies all at once, thereby enabling them all to be processed at once, thereby approximating the effect of eating a source of "complete" protein, such as meat.

But hear Nathan Pritikin on this subject. In *The Pritikin Program for Diet and Exercise* (Grosset & Dunlap; 1979), he starts by declaring that "the best food sources for protein are grains, roots, vegetables, and fruits in an unrefined, minimally processed form"—the heart, in fact, of his Pritikin Diet. He proclaims them better sources of protein than animal proteins that have high levels of fat and cholesterol.

"*All* natural food grown contains *all* of the amino acids, 'essential' and 'nonessential,' in sufficient quantities to satisfy human requirements," he asserts. "To speak of 'superior' and 'inferior' protein is nonsense."

The nomenclature "complete" and "incomplete" for protein dates from a 1916 study done with rats. But, as Pritikin points out, humans and rats do not have the same nutritional needs; rat's milk contains eight times the amount of protein found in human milk.

The need for protein is to provide a positive balance of nitrogen—a chief component of protein foods—in the body. But tests have found that even white rice as a principal protein source for adults provided the necessary nitrogen balance.

Pritikin acknowledges that a diet that omitted meat altogether *might* lead to a vitamin B_{12} deficiency "after five or ten years on a strict vegetarian diet." Actually, B_{12} is found in all animal proteins including dairy foods and fish, and while the possibility of this deficiency—which can result in pernicious anemia—is much publicized, it seems remote for most people.

I have yet to meet an anemic vegetarian. One man who has followed a strict macrobiotic diet for thirteen years related how his father-in-law, on a traditional meat-eating diet, developed anemia. Macrobiotics teachers have their own theory about this, which has to do with the quality of the blood produced by eating various foods. They also suggest that foods commonly eaten in a macrobiotic diet, including seaweeds and some soy products, are sources of B_{12}.

In any case, it does seem likely that the danger of protein deficiencies has been somewhat, if not vastly, overrated in our culture, and that the fear of protein deficiencies has been reinforced by various sources who may not have the consumer's best interests at heart.

On the other hand, studies have been emerging for some time that show there are health problems associated with eating too much animal protein. Chief among these is the risk of consuming excess fats and cholesterol, since animal foods tend to be high in both. My own experience when I stopped eating red meat was surprising. I had read that I might expect to lose weight on making any major change in diet, but that the weight would come back when I adjusted to the new diet. As I left meat more and more out of my diet, people did indeed begin to compliment me on how much weight I had lost. The truth of the matter was that I had lost only about five pounds. What I had lost, apparently, was a layer of fat that had been with me for years.

Many athletes find that good-quality carbohydrates, rather

DID YOU KNOW? Vitamin B_{12}, which is needed to prevent anemia, is found not just in meat but in all animal proteins including dairy foods. Some soy products and seaweeds are used in macrobiotics as sources of B_{12}.

---

than traditional animal proteins, can be used to advantage as the center of their diet. Bill Walton, the vegetarian basketball player, is probably the most famous. Julie Brown, the Olympic marathon runner, is not a strict vegetarian, but makes whole grains and vegetables the mainstay of her diet.

Marcie Schwam, world-class marathon runner and holder of a number of national and world records, has been a runner for seventeen years and a vegetarian for twelve of those years. She eats some dairy food ("mostly cheese") and no other animal food, but gets her protein from plant sources, including soybeans. She says it is common for runners to eat no red meat, a fact that might surprise non-runners. Runners seek non-fatty foods to keep their bodies lean, and emphasize a high carbohydrate intake to replace the energy used up in running. Carbohydrates are also favored over meat as being more digestible.

For Schwam, not eating meat was a moral decision. She says that even an endurance athlete like herself finds there is no real need for it, with the numerous other sources of protein and iron available.

Another health hazard in eating meat is that of disease. Lappe, among others, has outlined the fearsome conditions in which our nation's beef, poultry and dairy foods are produced —the dirty, overcrowded pens, the birds with their feet grown around the wire mesh of their cages, the kinds of environments that would set the American Society for the Prevention of Cruelty to Animals screaming if pets were subjected to them. One antidote to these conditions is to feed the livestock antibiotics, and the antibiotics are passed on up the food chain to us, with who knows what results twenty years from now.

The results of one feeding practice have already been questioned by the government: fattening livestock more rapidly—for greater profit—by dosing them with hormones.

One hormone, diethylstilbesterol (DES), used in fattening cattle and sheep, was banned in 1979 by the FDA after a long

---

DID YOU KNOW? Protein is needed to provide a positive balance of nitrogen in the body. But tests found that even white rice provided the necessary nitrogen balance for adults.

---

battle. DES, a known human carcinogen, was routinely mixed with livestock feed or implanted surgically. It had been suspect since 1938, when lab tests with DES caused malignant tumors in animals. In the 1940s it was administered in large doses to pregnant women as a means of preventing miscarriages. By 1971, a statistically significant number of these women's daughters were showing up with rare cancers of the reproductive tract, including vaginal cancer. In September 1980, *Consumer Reports* reported that FDA evidence showed that 415,000 animals had been treated with DES, despite the 1979 ban, and 30,000 of those had been sold or otherwise consigned as food for humans.

More recently, doctors in Puerto Rico have reported alarming rates of sexual development in babies—the development of breasts and lactation—believed to be associated with the use of hormones in poultry feed.

Another reason for reducing our intake of animal protein is, of course, at the heart of Lappe's crusade against world hunger: the amount of food needed to produce meat for the tables of America that could go to feed a hungry world instead. If this argument moves you, it is only fair to point out that in America even more grain goes to produce alcoholic beverages.

It is likely that the gradual vegetarian, even if he gives up meat altogether, will still be consuming *much more protein* than he needs, if he eats at all sensibly. One study shows the following set of comparisons: 3.5 ounces of chicken provides

18.2 grams of protein, as compared with 34.1 grams in the same amount of soybeans; beef contributes 16.9 grams; cow's milk furnishes 3.5 grams. And vegetable foods also provide something that animal proteins can't—an outstanding source of slow-burning carbohydrates, with minimum fat.

THE STAFF OF LIFE

The real mainstay of diets the world over—diets through history, the Pritikin Diet, and the vegetarian diet—is, of course, the carbohydrate.

Carbohydrates include starches (complex carbohydrates) and sugars (simple carbohydrates). Meat contains no carbohydrates.

The carbohydrates we are especially interested in are the complex carbohydrates found in natural, unprocessed grains, fruits and vegetables. These are the ideal fuel for the human body's metabolism because they are digested slowly and steadily—unlike the simple carbohydrates such as refined sugar, which break down almost immediately, flooding the bloodstream and brain with glucose, creating a sugar "high."

The complex carbohydrates are also more easily digested than fatty foods and proteins, without the latter's residue of wastes. Complex carbohydrates are the body's "clean energy," leaving as waste only carbon dioxide and water, both of which the body casts off routinely.

People who are weight-conscious have been programmed

Did You Know? A comparison shows 3.5 ounces of chicken provides 18.2 grams of protein, while the same amount of soybeans yields 34.1 grams; beef, 16.9 grams; cow's milk, 3.5 grams.

to think of starches as synonymous with weight gain. The truth is, in our culture, we seldom eat even the best-quality carbohydrate foods without loading them with fats, salt and/ or refined sugar. Vegetables are buttered, cereals are laced with sugar and cream, salads are "dressed," fruits are baked into gooey pies with fatty crusts; in short, our carbohydrates rarely come to us in unadulterated form. While it is not necessary to be spartan, unless one's health has already deteriorated to the point of emergency, it is certainly prudent to bring one's eating more into line with the realities of what's good for the body. And what's good for the body is simpler foods than what most Americans eat.

In pursuit of these foods, we naturally may begin to think of the grain foods as our forebears did. The bread that was the staff of life was certainly made of coarse, barely refined flours—oats, barley, wheat, buckwheat, legumes, rice—probably with some grit from the millstone mixed in. We read a lot about oat cakes and barley cakes in medieval Europe; in the Orient, rice was a staple, and noodles were perhaps being invented; in the Middle East, millet was a popular grain. In our own time, until the advent of the health food store, our vocabulary of grains had become miserably impoverished. Now we must consciously expand it, relearning the uses of the major grains. This is especially important to the person who is contemplating a more strictly vegetarian diet, to introduce variety.

The grains in their whole form may be used as cooked cereal for breakfast, or as the chief ingredient of a main dish for lunches and dinners. We are most familiar with rice, but millet can be used interchangeably; it is a lighter and sweeter grain with a pleasing texture. Modestly refined grain products like kasha (from buckwheat), bulgur wheat and couscous can also be substituted for rice.

Legumes, especially beans and lentils, and nuts also become integral parts of casseroles, non-meat loaves, and other entrées. Flour made from whole grains can be used to make bread that is almost a meal in itself, or can go into homemade noodles and pasta. Soy products can be the star attraction in a main dish like tofu shish kebab, or function behind the scenes as in tempeh in vegetarian chili, or soy flour in bread.

As explained in Stage One, it is important to keep grains and nuts properly stored away from heat. The more they are processed, the more subject they are to rancidity, because of their oil content, unless a stabilizing factor like hydrogenation is introduced. In American homes, which tend to be overheated, the simplest procedure is to refrigerate anything that may be subject to rancidity. I refrigerate all flour, corn meal, bran, wheat germ, sesame seeds, nut meats and nut butters, as well as oils, of course. I store rice, legumes, kasha, barley, bulgur wheat and millet away from heat and light in airtight containers in a cupboard.

In comparing the relative merits of grains and legumes, it is perhaps unnecessary to mention that soybeans provide "complete" protein—all the "essential" amino acids. Soy products have gotten a great deal of publicity because of their high protein content, and are a mainstay of many packaged preparations at the health food store. If you are concerned about getting enough protein, you will want to think about baking with soy flour and exploring other soy products, like tofu, miso and tamari sauce.

In addition, there are other characteristics of the various grains that are worth noting. Brown rice is the grain highest in B vitamins; buckwheat is said to be high in vitamin E. Wheat is valuable in baking because it is the grain highest in gluten, necessary for the bread's rising. It is also highest in protein. Corn has the highest sugar content, and oats are relatively high in fat. Millet is the only alkaline grain, according to Naboru Muramoto, and is high in protein as well. Rye is a secondary grain in baking in our culture, while barley is usually used in its whole form, in soups. An additional grain, triticale, is a hybrid of rye and wheat. Relatively low in gluten, it is used for flour and in some cereal mixtures.

Besides the protein-rich grains and legumes, all fruits and vegetables contain carbohydrates in varying degrees. These are also our best natural sources of vitamins and minerals and a valuable source of fiber as well.

Especially rich in carbohydrates are potatoes, the winter squashes and pumpkin, and the sweet fruits, including bananas, grapes and raisins, dried dates and figs. These are followed by mildly starchy vegetables, including cauliflower, beets and carrots, and by other fruits: apples, pears, peaches, apricots, plums, cherries, berries and citrus fruits.

VITAMINS AND MINERALS

Fruits and vegetables are probably better known to us as the bearers of vital minerals and vitamins, which our school texts assured us would be supplied (somewhat magically, it seemed to me) if we diligently ate our daily helpings of citrus fruit and green and yellow vegetables.

This, like much else in life, turns out to be less simple than it sounded; no mention was made, in those schoolbook examples, of growing conditions, fruits being picked unripe, shipping and prolonged storage, or loss of vitamins through cooking or other processing.

It is not the purpose of this book to prescribe vitamin or mineral therapy. But I do suggest that it helps to be educated on a basic level about the body's needs and about what foods provide what nutrients.

One problem with determining one's own needs is that no two bodies are the same in their chemical make-up, any more than in any other way. The U.S. Recommended Daily Allowances, or the National Academy of Science's Dietary Allowances—both abbreviated as RDAs—are just that: recommended, on the basis of laboratory studies, for a hypothetical average American.

A second problem is that we—and sometimes the experts

—tend to approach our bodies like inanimate objects. When it comes to their care and feeding, we treat them like machines, to be gassed up every so often and given periodic tune-ups. The trouble is that the body, unlike a machine, never stops working, and that, unlike a machine, it acts upon every substance that enters it.

So in becoming aware of RDAs and the like, we should not assume that what will work best is simply to chuck all the RDAs of various vital substances down our throats once a day, or think that to be knowledgeable about certain statistics is to understand how the body functions—how we live.

The fact is that there is much that even the experts do not know about how we live, and that RDAs are just one way—the method chosen by Western science in the twentieth century—to speak of the transmutation of energy that keeps us alive. So we should know what they are, as a point of reference, but our curiosity about what is nutritionally good for us should not stop there. The great unknown quantity in all of this is our digestive system. The point, after all, is not how much protein or vitamin A or potassium or whatever is *in*gested—but how much is *di*gested, assimilated by the body. The body can function splendidly if it is in good working order, with a healthy supply of the friendly bacteria necessary to digestion at work in the intestines; a bloodstream that is not cluttered up with fat; lungs that are not so polluted that they are unable to absorb the requisite oxygen; and a liver that is not loaded down with toxins. A healthy body can process the valuable substances and excrete wastes without delay; it can also manufacture vital substances on its own. An overworked body may simply become more overburdened, particularly if we feed it carelessly.

Let us consider some of the ways we may expect our altered eating habits to affect our daily intake of some of the essential nutrients we need for health.

Without meat, there is not the automatic consumption of large amounts of protein, and we accordingly look for it in other places. In a more or less meatless diet, we can also expect a reduced sodium intake. This will not be a problem for most people, and may even be a benefit. But we will have to find other sources for the B vitamins, of which the best known source—regrettably—is liver.

In the absence of meat, there is a natural tendency to substitute dairy foods. But we want to be careful of these, too, since many are high in fat content. And some vegetarians may wish to give up animal foods altogether. So we must be aware of alternative sources of calcium and vitamin A, two key nutrients derived from milk products.

On the plus side, fresh vegetables that have not been overcooked will make up an increasing portion of the diet, and they are variously rich in vitamins A and C, so that natural sources of these will be added automatically. An increased diet of whole grains, nuts and seeds will mean a supply of vitamin E almost certainly very much superior to that of the standard American diet. Some B vitamins will be supplied in whole grains, and more in dairy foods and fish. For added sources rich in B vitamins, soy foods like miso and tempeh are excellent; and the macrobiotic tea, bancha, plus all of the seaweeds, provide calcium, which is also found in sesame seeds.

The soy foods and other macrobiotic products will be introduced later in more detail. I mention them now only to

---

DID YOU KNOW? The herb comfrey is rich in calcium and potassium, and its leaves are high in vitamins A and C. It also contains vitamin B_{12} and the amino acid lysine, not commonly found outside animal foods, plus niacin, pantothenic acid, choline, and vitamins B_1, B_2, D and E.

point out that there are many alternatives—some of them quite surprising—for the essential nutrients. We really need not be locked in by a fear of not getting enough protein, calcium, vitamin B_{12} or whatever.

There are other good sources of the B vitamins, and they are important especially because the B vitamins are water soluble and are constantly washing out of our systems. This also is true of vitamin C, but not of vitamins A, D, E or K, which are fat soluble and accumulate in our fatty tissues. Yeast, of which debittered versions are available in health food stores, is one of the richest non-meat sources of B vitamins. It does have a distinctive taste that is best disguised, by dissolving it thoroughly in fruit, tomato or V-8 juice, or by adding it to any dish that has a strong flavor of its own. If you are not going to use soy products as sources of vitamin B, get into the habit of adding yeast to any legume or tomato dishes, including soups, lasagnes, and non-meat loaves. Use a little at first and experiment with adding a little more if no one complains.

Some people find yeast difficult to digest, and intestinal gas may result unless and until healthy intestinal flora are established. Yogurt and the cultured or fermented soy products provide these flora, along with many of the B vitamins. Another surprising source of B vitamins, including B_{12}, is the herb comfrey. A friend of mine tells of watching wild deer walk right into her front yard in a rural suburb of New York City, just to eat the leaves of the large comfrey plant that grows there. Comfrey is rich in calcium and potassium, and its leaves are high in vitamin A and C. It also contains the amino acid lysine, another substance not commonly found outside animal foods; vitamins B_1, B_2, D, E; niacin; pantothenic acid; and choline. Comfrey is available in health food stores in root and leaf form, for making into tea. It has a rather dull, earthy flavor, and is best mixed with a mint or carob-flavored tea, with a little honey or milk.

Other herb teas are also high in valuable nutrients—vitamin C in rose hips; vitamins A and E in alfalfa, which also offers protein and B vitamins; and, in ginseng, a substance that stimulates the metabolism of vitamins and minerals and has been reported effective in countering vitamin B deficiencies.

Then there are the minerals we need for good health. Besides calcium, these are chiefly potassium, sodium and magnesium. The balance of these minerals enables the flow of nutrients and oxygen into cells by osmosis, and the removal of wastes and toxins through the cell walls into the bloodstream, which transports them to the excretory organs for disposal. The minerals, properly balanced, actually help pass nutrient-bearing body fluids into the cells and pull wastes out. Calcium and magnesium, for instance, must be balanced in a ratio of 2 to 1; and the body needs 800–1,200 milligrams of calcium daily. Calcium taken in excess can induce a magnesium deficiency, while too much magnesium can cause lethargy, drowsiness and even coma. Calcium, of course, is richly supplied by dairy foods, while magnesium is found in nuts, tofu, dark leafy greens and seaweed. So a vegetarian diet may actually mean a healthier balance of these minerals. Magnesium, however, is contained in laxatives and antacids, and could be oversupplied in people who use them (one good reason not to).

Similarly potassium and sodium must be balanced—5,000 milligrams of potassium per 2,100 milligrams of sodium (the amount in 1 teaspoon of table salt). Since sodium is richly

---

DID YOU KNOW? Besides calcium, minerals needed for health include potassium, sodium and magnesium. The balance of these minerals enables the flow of nutrients and oxygen into cells by osmosis and the removal of wastes through the cell walls.

---

supplied in meats, table salt and salty foods, there is no lack of it in modern American diets, especially at the fast-food end of the spectrum. Potassium, meanwhile, is found in fruits, vegetables, whole grains, nuts and seaweed, as well as in meats. Potassium cannot be retained unless the supply of magnesium is adequate, which is a further way in which the minerals interlock.

All of these nutrients can be supplied amply to our bodies if we eat a balanced vegetarian diet free of the excesses that are so available all around us. As we contemplate a shift to a non-meat-eating cuisine, we must envision the component parts of the new diet that will replace the more familiar sources of needed nutrients. Our balance of vital minerals, calcium, potassium, sodium and magnesium may actually be improved by a more vegetarian diet.

BODY LANGUAGE

If health is a primary or even secondary goal in revising your eating style, your curiosity should lead you into a more intimate dialogue with your own body, which will help tell you what foods to eat. We already know the experience of our bodies telling us what *not* to eat. When we're sick, we voluntarily and even automatically become finicky, eat lightly, perhaps even go on a near-liquid fast. We accept the body's wisdom in dealing with a cold or minor infection.

As we become more attuned to our diet, the body is prepared to give us more subtle clues about what it really needs. I am not talking about a craving for ice cream that springs from a well-developed sweet tooth. I am talking about a constant state of good health: clear skin, good energy levels throughout the day, and the absence of headaches, sniffles and intestinal disorders.

Your body will tell you these things, of course, only if you let it have a clear channel free of static. You can't possibly hear what it has to say about acorn squash if your nervous system is chattering away about chocolate, alcohol, tobacco, sugar and caffeine.

That does not mean that you can never consume any extreme foods. But it does mean that you can't be addicted to any of them. If you think you need any of them as often as once a day, we are talking about a habit that must be laid aside before further communication with the body can take place. Then, on occasions when you do partake of these extreme foods, you will quickly notice your body telling you that's what they are.

In the typical American diet, the chances are you are getting more than enough protein, fats, simple carbohydrates and sodium and rather less than enough of certain vitamins and of complex carbohydrates. Perhaps you're eating out a lot and getting soggy, overcooked vegetables from which the vitamin A has long since departed. Or perhaps you don't really bother to fix vegetables at home—especially the yellow or dark green and leafy ones. Again there's a possible lack of vitamin A, which is aggravated by working under artificial light. On the other hand, perhaps you're drinking lots of milk and getting your vitamin A quota that way.

Nutritional therapy is a vast subject. If you have reason to think that your health is below par and has been for some time, a nutritional analysis and diagnosis by an expert—a qualified nutritionist or a medical doctor who is versed in nutrition—may be in order. But a reliance on simpler foods simply prepared may put you into a better state of health all by itself. Certainly simple preparation of unprocessed foods will at least guarantee that your body has a chance to get maximum good out of them.

THE FAT OF THE LAND

And speaking of preparation brings us to the subject of fats and oil, those closet villains of the kitchen. Anyone who has gone on a low-fat diet knows to his sorrow that food as we know it is not to be found in the realm of the fat-free. Instead, there's salad without dressing, bread without butter, no french fries, no creamy sauces. A culinary wasteland.

It's not necessary for most people to go that far to reach a level of sanity in eating, but it is good to recognize the prevalence of fat—hidden or obvious—in the American diet, and to deal with it creatively, to lessen our own fat intake if need be.

The effect of fat in our systems is to clog the circulation, in combination with cholesterol, forming deposits of plaque along the insides of the blood vessels. Fats also impede the blood itself in one of its major functions—that of carrying oxygen to all the cells in the body, including of course those in the brain. Fats are not easily digested, and in the bloodstream they form a film around the oxygen-carrying red blood cells. Fat cells in animals also are the repositories of chemical toxins and wastes, which are passed up the food chain from the lowest level to the highest, increasing in concentration all the way.

Fats are not an efficient food from a standpoint of digestion. People who shift away from a diet of animal foods are naturally going to eat fewer saturated fats and probably fewer fats in general. But it is important to remember that most dairy foods, and eggs, are also rich in fat and cholesterol. Dairy foods can certainly substitute for meat in entrées, but they must be used judiciously. And it should be remembered, too, in contemplating your intake of fats, that the unsaturated fats—the oil in the salad dressing and in the stir-fry—are still fats, even though they are more easily handled by the body. There are a lot of uses of fats that need not be automatic, like butter on vegetables, cream in sauces and soups, and fat in cooking. Unsaturated oil can be used to garnish vegetables, yogurt can substitute for sweet or sour cream in most recipes, and for those especially concerned with limiting fat intake, low-fat milk and cheeses can be substituted routinely in recipes. You may also want to begin exploring tofu as a substitute for cheese in recipes.

Whatever your reasons for exploring a vegetarian cuisine, a decision to stop eating meat altogether is a kind of middle step between a traditional diet and the stricter vegetarian diets. People in this middle ground often describe themselves as lacto-ovo-vegetarians because they continue to eat eggs and dairy foods. Some people at this point also continue to eat fish, as do some who follow a relatively stricter macrobiotic diet. But at this point, it is important to try to view plant foods—grains, vegetables and fruits—as the legitimate centerpiece of meals.

STAGE TWO: MIDPOINT

You are still eating fish in Stage Two, but you have stopped eating poultry almost entirely. You are using more dairy foods, grains, legumes, nuts and seeds as centerpieces for your meals. A look at a day's sample menus illustrates the benefits and potential pitfalls of eating more vegetables and less meat. This is a day of fairly light eating (about 1,500 calories), chosen to show you what your minimum menus might give you in the way of essential nutrients.

Breakfast: 1 cup of cooked oatmeal, with an apple sliced and cooked into it, 8 ounces of yogurt and 4 ounces milk.

Lunch: a pita pocket stuffed with a half cup of hummus and a cup of shredded salad (lettuce, cabbage, carrots, green pepper); a few cherry tomatoes; 2 ounces of raisins.

Dinner: Garden Vegetable Soup (this could be left over from a previous dinner) and Shells and Broccoli (see Index for recipes).

TAKE NOTE:

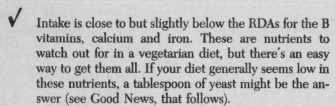

✓ Intake is close to but slightly below the RDAs for the B vitamins, calcium and iron. These are nutrients to watch out for in a vegetarian diet, but there's an easy way to get them all. If your diet generally seems low in these nutrients, a tablespoon of yeast might be the answer (see Good News, that follows).

✓ A day of light eating can be low in carbohydrate grams as well. This one provides about two-thirds the RDA for women and about one-half the RDA for men. This is probably of little concern generally, since a day of heavier eating will balance it out, but people who seek

a high-carbohydrate diet will want to note the Good
News that follows.

GOOD NEWS:

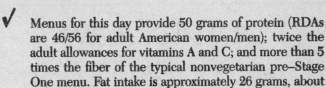 Menus for this day provide 50 grams of protein (RDAs
are 46/56 for adult American women/men); twice the
adult allowances for vitamins A and C; and more than 5
times the fiber of the typical nonvegetarian pre–Stage
One menu. Fat intake is approximately 26 grams, about
one-sixth the intake of the nonvegetarian menu.

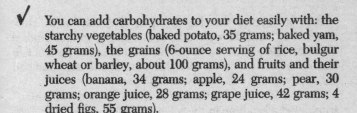 One ounce of debittered yeast, available in health food
stores, provides the following: 79 calories, 11 protein
grams, 10 carbohydrate grams and .3 fat gram. It also
furnishes more than twice the RDA of vitamin B_1; more
than half the RDA of vitamin B_2; one-fourth the RDA of
vitamin B_6; one-sixth the RDA of calcium; and half the
RDA of iron for adult men or one-third the RDA for
women. Add yeast by the teaspoon to juice, soup, and
legume dishes including hummus and peanut butter.

✓ You can add carbohydrates to your diet easily with: the
starchy vegetables (baked potato, 35 grams; baked yam,
45 grams), the grains (6-ounce serving of rice, bulgur
wheat or barley, about 100 grams), and fruits and their
juices (banana, 34 grams; apple, 24 grams; pear, 30
grams; orange juice, 28 grams; grape juice, 42 grams; 4
dried figs, 55 grams).

EIGHT

AN ACCIDENT
OF
GEOGRAPHY

*I*t is important to remember that virtually all of our eating habits are thrust upon us by society. Human beings eat every conceivable kind of food, and it is only an accident of birth and geography that determines whether we eat fruits or roots, grasshoppers or filet mignon, bland kasha or spicy curry.

It is our society that has given us "Fat City" and "How sweet it is," and their attendant ills. Among various studies that have come down on the American diet rather hard of late is one that focuses on the idea that you not only are what you eat, but you also are what you don't eat.

"Eating less may be the key to living beyond 100 years," trumpeted a headline in the science section of *The New York Times* (June 6, 1982). The article by Jane Brody reported studies with laboratory rats at the University of Texas that showed that cutting the protein intake of the animals by one half significantly lengthened their lives, as did reducing their calorie intake to sixty percent of normal. (Meats, while they contain no carbohydrates, are high in both fats and calories.) The same article reported that studies done at Sloan-Kettering Cancer Center in New York showed that lowering the fat composition of the diets of laboratory mice reduced their risk of developing cancer and diseases related to immunological deficiencies. Putting them on a low-protein diet reduced the toll of the aging process on their immune systems.

A similar study conducted at the University of California at Los Angeles by Dr. Roy Walford, a pathologist and expert on aging, concluded: "Long-term undernutrition is thus far the only method we know of that retards aging and extends the maximum life span of warm-blooded mammals."

For the time being, however, let us focus on what we do eat. The person who quits eating meat altogether is faced with some very real concerns about what to eat instead.

You have perhaps already looked at the options and decided that dairy foods and eggs are too high in cholesterol and fat to be a really helpful substitute. And you are perhaps not all that familiar with the other options.

Several things are worth noting right away. First, while it is true that many dairy foods are high in cholesterol and/or fat, this is not universally true. Second, you are eliminating a lot of potential fat and cholesterol from your diet by not eating meat, and can perhaps work out a diet that includes judicious use of milk, cheese and eggs. Third, many otherwise strict vegetarians do continue to include fish in their diets, so that may be an option for you.

But it is also time to be exploring grains and legumes more fully, and among these are soy and other products that have long been mainstays of the Oriental macrobiotic diet, but have only recently become widely available in this country.

It is only fair to say that many of these foods look and taste somewhat strange at first; some of them you may not even like—too bland, slightly bitter, uninteresting texture. But try them anyway. They are wonderfully nutritious without offering any drawbacks in terms of your health—an oblique way of saying they're *good* for you. And they can be incorporated into a number of very tasty dishes that are in the mainstream of Western traditional cuisines, or not far from it, so that you can enjoy them without resistance. Of course, ultimately you do get used to them and come to appreciate them in their unadulterated form, if that is your goal.

For the time being, though, we are talking about finding good sources of some of these basic ingredients and incorporating them into conventional dishes. Remember, as we go along, that it doesn't have to be forever. It doesn't hurt to try, and you can always return to an earlier stage at any point.

This is also a good time to think about upgrading sources of other ingredients. You may not feel it's necessary, for the time being or for the foreseeable future. Or you may have already decided it's time to seek a source of organic vegetables, raw milk and cheese, fertilized eggs. These steps, at least initially, will probably be more time-consuming and expensive than just obtaining your groceries at the supermarket. But they can be incorporated into your daily or weekly routine so that they become just that—routine.

WHERE TO BUY IT

At this point you are going to have to weigh economy and convenience against your own perceptions of quality. There seems little question that the flour products you buy at a health food store are better quality (providing they are fresh) than what you get at the supermarket. And the health food store has a greater variety of flour (rye, stone-ground corn meal or wheat flour). And in other areas the health food store also offers either more variety—in dried beans, rice, soy products; or better quality—peanut butter that's not hydrogenated, cold-pressed oils, raw honey; or products you often can't get elsewhere—whole wheat pasta, granola without sugar in it, yogurt with live cultures.

As for fresh produce, there is really no way short of laboratory testing to know how much pesticide is contained in a particular carrot. At best, you can grow it yourself or buy it from someone whose growing conditions you are able to observe. Not all health food stores carry fresh produce, but those that do are an expensive alternative to the grocery store.

In deciding what kind of strategy you are going to follow to improve your diet in this stage, I think it can't hurt to start buying most of your grain products at the health food store. You will want to find a store that is clean and where there is enough customer traffic to insure a fairly quick turnover of perishables. In the interests of one-stop shopping, you should try to find a health food store that also stocks a fair amount of macrobiotic supplies, including miso, tofu and seaweed. This may take some looking—and in the process you will find that all health food stores are not indeed equal. Some are franchises that actually belong to health food chains, and while they may offer high quality, their selection may also be limited. It is well worth getting to know the individual manager so that you can make special requests. If necessary, try new stores until you find one that meets your needs.

There are several other sources that can be very valuable. If your local health food stores doesn't stock the staples you want, you may find an Oriental grocery that does. A minor drawback here is that all the labeling information may be in Japanese, in which case you'll just have to ask for things by name and put up with a certain degree of trial and error.

Other sources of supply are worth pursuing: a good fish market or poultry farm; a dairy or goat farm that sells its products, perhaps including certified raw milk; a farm that sells organic produce and/or organic poultry and fertilized eggs; or simply a local farm stand where the produce is fresher and perhaps less treated for uniform appearance.

Another good source, which may lead you to all of the above and should certainly save you money, is a food co-op. You may find one by word of mouth or through local or national publications (including *East-West Journal* and

Mother Earth News). If you join one, you save money and you gain more power over what you buy.

WHAT TO BUY

What you are doing this time around is simply refining the shopping list you developed in Stage One.

In the health food store, try the short-grain and medium-grain varieties of rice, as well as the long-grain kind usually sold in supermarkets. Think about buying millet as well, to be used as a rice substitute, especially in Middle Eastern dishes, or cooked in with the rice. There's also bulgur wheat, a partly processed wheat product that is used in Tabbouleh Salad and can also be used instead of rice. Kasha is a similar partly processed grain, but is made from buckwheat. Both bulgur and kasha have the advantage of cooking quickly—10 to 15 minutes—and so are handy when you're in a hurry.

The legumes are probably near the grains, so look them over while you're there. You may find several varieties of lentil besides the greenish-brown ones sold in the supermarket. And, in addition to the familiar beans—kidney, pinto and navy—you may find black "turtle" beans, chick-peas and aduki (or azuki) beans. The black beans are a staple of Hispanic cooking and are commonly served with rice, often rice cooked with saffron to make it yellow. These beans also make a delicious Black Bean Soup. Chick-peas (also known as

DID YOU KNOW? Aduki beans are the least fatty of all beans and the most digestible—their low fat content minimizes the discomfort for which legumes are notorious. The aduki is also quicker-cooking than other beans.

garbanzo beans) are a mainstay of Middle Eastern cooking, where they are often ground to a flour or paste to form a principal ingredient in a dish like Falafel or Hummus.

Aduki beans are the least fatty of all beans, and are an important addition to your diet for that reason. They provide superior nutrition and are more digestible than the other beans; among their other virtues, their low fat content makes for less discomfort from gas. Aduki beans, because of their low fat, also tend to cook up drier, and must be watched to see they don't burn. It also helps to cook them in extra water, adding it along the way, so that there is liquid, or "pot liquor," left at the end to allay the dryness. Adukis also cook somewhat more quickly than the larger beans, although not as quickly as lentils. If you can't get them at a health food store, they are usually available at Oriental groceries.

Also with the grains and beans you may find whole sesame seeds. These can also sometimes be bought at Oriental, Middle Eastern or Italian groceries. They are the essential ingredient of a Japanese condiment called *gomasio*, which is essentially a mild and digestible salt dish. Sesame seeds are also good toasted, to be used in salads, cereal, stir-fry, vegetable dishes, non-meat loaf—whenever you think of them, in short. Why bother, given that they, like nuts, are expensive? Well, if you are concerned about protein, they are or can be part of the great protein balancing act. And if you're feeling secure about protein, they are still important for the *gomasio*, which, as we'll see, is a good way of getting our salt flavor and some oil too without taxing our digestive systems unduly.

And speaking of nuts and expense, look for sunflower seeds on the grain and bean shelf, too—they're a substitute for the more expensive pine nuts (pignoli) in pesto, and are an ingredient of homemade granola, too.

Also important at the health food store is the pasta aisle. Buy some whole wheat products and try those made with Jerusalem artichoke as well—they contain less wheat but taste like the real thing. Personal favorites are Westbrae's

Veggie Bows—whole wheat and vegetable macaroni elbows that are delicious in casseroles—and DeBoles' Jerusalem-artichoke-and-spinach pasta, a brilliant green, elegant in any dish.

As for flour, get your unbleached here, and corn meal too if you use it, for basic cooking. Then, if you're a baker already or planning to try your hand at yeast breads, look at the other flours they have—rye, soy, whole wheat. Whole wheat flour is handy to add to quick breads, as well as pancakes and pies.

TAKING STOCK OF WHAT'S GOOD TO EAT

If we are going to eat less animal food, an effort should be made to insure that what we do eat is of the best quality.

What do we mean by the best quality? One way of looking at it is that what is least processed is best.

Certainly at the basic level this is easy enough to verify: plain yogurt is more completely digestible and better for you than yogurt loaded with sugar and chemicals. And why buy the latter, which is more expensive, when plain yogurt can become any flavor you want with the addition of a little cooked fruit?

Beyond this level, we are almost invariably talking about trade-offs of quality against convenience and cost.

"Organic" or fertilized chicken eggs represent less human tampering and in this sense are less "processed." But they cost more and you have to go to a health food store or a farm to get them. Is it worth it? This is one of the trade-offs you have to consider, and here are some others:

■ Raw milk has been declared superior to pasteurized-homogenized by various nutritionists. In cost and convenience, it presents the same problems as the eggs. Also it sours quickly, although it can still be used. Additionally, there is the somewhat remote but still real chance of a contact with undulant fever through milk that has not been pasteurized. An outbreak of it was reported in southern New Jersey cattle herds in 1982. A rare disease in humans, it can be recurrent once contracted, and produces symptoms like flu.

■ In considering dairy foods, it has been proven that goat's milk is more digestible by humans than cow's milk. It is recommended when an allergy to cow's milk has been diagnosed, and it is closer in quality to human milk. It is also much harder to find than cow's milk. Additionally, there is sometimes the goat taste, which carries over into products like yogurt and cheese. Is it worth it to go to the trouble of finding the goat milk or cheese, and then getting used to the taste? It is if you have decided you can't live without dairy food but are unable to tolerate cow's milk. If you decide to try goat's milk, do yourself the favor of buying it as fresh as possible. Goat's cheese—often called by its French name, *chèvre*—is available in gourmet cheese shops, and represents an easier way to get used to the flavor. Feta cheese also is made from goat's milk.

■ Is it worth the extra expense and trouble to buy totally unprocessed cheese—that which continues to age—at special cheese stores? Or to buy rennetless cheese—that which does not contain the animal-based coagulant rennet—at the health food store? Or, if you are still eating some poultry, to buy "organic" chicken—that which has been raised on feed free of hormones, antibiotics and chemical additives—at a farm or health food store?

It depends on the state of your health, your mind and your purse. For me, health stepped in to dictate. I had continuing, if generally mild, hay-fever allergies that were aggravated by the consumption of mucus-forming foods, which virtually everyone including the medical establishment agrees include dairy foods. So I had a real incentive to cut down on these and to look for alternatives—and that led me to examine the stricter vegetarian diets.

Your state of mind might be shaped by things like how much time and energy you have to spend on foraging for food, and for how many and what kind of eaters. Maybe you will want to make one or two items your priority; or perhaps you will decide that the items available on the mass market are generally O.K. Or you may decide that, for the same amount of trouble, you could be living on a completely vegetable, fruit and grain diet.

The Stage Two recipes assume that most people will gravitate to a diet that includes dairy foods, and there may be a good reason for that, as we will see in Stage Three. But they also show how we can begin to introduce the soy foods discussed in Chapter 9, and lean away from the richer dairy dishes.

Two further thoughts: If the state of your purse is a consideration, do remember that while high-quality foods are an extra expense, you are also saving a tremendous amount of money if you are not routinely buying meats, coffee, snack foods, soda pop and commercially made desserts. And if your health improves, you are saving on over-the-counter drugs—and maybe even prescriptions.

WHAT ABOUT ALLERGIES?

The most common food allergies are to wheat, milk (and related products), eggs and chocolate. What does this mean for a vegetarian?

Obviously, if you're a person with food allergies, it means that you may be despairing of a diet based on grains. Don't. If wheat is your special demon, there are ways of working around it. But equally important is knowing what the allergy does, why we have it, and how we may get rid of it.

An allergy or an adverse reaction resembling an allergy may be triggered by an abnormal amount of stress. Allergies and allergy-like reactions have become increasingly commonplace in the twentieth century. It is notable that we are living in an era of high stress just from our environment. There's noise pollution, water pollution, air pollution and the emotional stress brought on by trying to keep up in a high-speed, high-technology environment permeated by mass media and an attendant stream of stressful news that warns us of threats to our very survival: news of wars, the economy, and the environment itself.

Rather than dose ourselves with antihistamines, we may be able to correct the situation with diet. In the case of really severe allergies, outside help may be needed to relieve years of accumulated stress. It has even been suggested that allergies may get started in infants who are fed formula instead of breast-fed, because they miss the total nutrition provided—and individualized—in mother's milk. In severe cases of allergy it may be appropriate to seek relief by consulting a chiropractor, nutritionist, or shiatsu therapist, or try some other form of accredited natural therapy to help restore the body's own defenses. But serious attention to one's own patterns of stressful behavior may also provide many of the answers.

Stress is categorized as physical, chemical, thermal and emotional. Physical stress may result from overwork, lack of sleep, injury and illness. The antidote usually is rest. Thermal stress is a reflection of the fact that coping with extremes of temperature puts a strain on the body, and while this does not mean we must retreat into a thermostatically controlled environment, it does mean we should use common sense about dress and exposure to extremes of climate.

Emotional stress is something each person must judge. The most uncontrollable portion usually comes from the workplace. One nice side effect of more balanced dietary habits—minus the caffeine and sugar and tobacco and such—is increased tranquility.

Chemical stress includes any poison, however subtle—pollution, toxins in the workplace, and unnatural or extreme food substances. These include food additives, refined foods that are consequently out of balance with nature, and the extreme substances—alcohol, tobacco, sugar, caffeine, chocolate.

What, you may want to know, does all of this have to do with an allergy to wheat, if wheat is one of the natural substances we are touting? Simply that denaturalized wheat is contained in many refined foods, which may account for its prominent place on the list of allergy-making foods. And second, once the normal balance of the body is restored through elimination of undue stress, people sometimes find that they are no longer allergic and may resume limited contact with previously taboo substances.

Jonathan Wright, *Prevention* magazine's resident M.D., has this to say about allergies in *Dr. Wright's Book of Nutritional Therapy* (Rodale Press; 1979): "Your body's cells are adapted to the same foods humans have eaten for three or four million years. . . . The earliest evidence of farming and animal domestication . . . dates from about 8000 to 15,000 B.C.

DID YOU KNOW? A diet for people with allergies to wheat, eggs and cow's milk can include wheat-free breads from a health food store; oats for cereal; Japanese buckwheat noodles and a variety of Oriental rice noodles. Tofu can replace eggs and cheese in some recipes, and goat's milk, juice or water may substitute for cow's milk.

"Now ten thousand years seems like a terribly long time to you and me. But in perspective, it's only about one-half per cent of the total time of human existence. . . .

"So it shouldn't be much of a surprise that foods only recently introduced into the human diet as a result of farming and animal domestication should frequently be the source of symptoms or diseases. Wheat, corn, eggs, milk: these and many other natural and wholesome foods are perfectly capable of causing illness in persons whose body chemistry isn't suited to them."

Dr. Wright neglects to mention the over-abundance of meat available to those who domesticate animals on a massive scale, as we do in twentieth-century America—but we can add that to the list.

The macrobiotics specialists emphasize that correct diet may banish your allergies. But meanwhile, what are you supposed to do if wheat is your allergy?

In general cooking, use other flours as a thickening agent. Baking without wheat flour is a problem in yeast-raised breads, since the wheat gluten acts as part of the rising agent. You may be able to purchase wheat-free breads at a health food store or to special order them. In the realm of breakfast cereals, wheat is not a must, since oats are the base of the main cereals. And in pasta, the picture is not nearly as bleak as you'd expect—there is *soba*, a Japanese buckwheat noodle, and a variety of rice noodles, obtainable in Oriental food stores. And, assuming your allergy comes under control as you leave refined foods behind, the pastas made with spinach and Jerusalem-artichoke flour contain a smaller amount of wheat and may prove practicable.

Dairy-food allergies are a real nuisance in a culture brought up on the ideal of three glasses of cow's milk a day. Of course, cow's milk and the eggs we eat are both, as noted, foods we've tampered with—the eggs aren't fertilized, and the milk is pasteurized, homogenized and fortified to a fare-thee-well. But in any case, cow's milk is a food the human system doesn't digest well.

This is not the tragedy it might seem. It is inconvenient though not impossible to do without eggs in baking and numerous recipes. But for cow's milk there are plenty of substitutes, ranging from goat's milk to juice to water. In lieu of cheeses and eggs, tofu can be substituted in many recipes, though admittedly neither it nor goat cheese tastes like what we're used to.

For those with the special problem of allergies, *The Egg-Free, Milk-Free, Wheat-Free Cookbook* (Harper & Row; 1982) by Becky Hamrick and S. L. Wiesenfeld, M.D.s, may offer more interim help in getting weaned from wheat, dairy foods and chemical additives. Allergy sufferers may also be interested to know that a strict macrobiotic diet may be followed and enjoyed without ever using wheat (or, of course, dairy foods).

SO TRY IT

I have been talking about the "accident of birth" that dropped us down in a meat-eating, wheat-eating, milk-guzzling culture where all kinds of stresses abound. Of course, we are also lucky to be living in what is probably the technologically most advanced culture in human history, where our choice of food—and so many other things—can be infinite. What we are seeking is a balance for our bodies, and the simple way in the midst of plenty.

For those with allergies and for those who simply want to expand their vegetarian vocabulary, there is one food we really haven't discussed, whose uses are so many and whose qualities are so special that it really deserves a chapter to itself. It is of course the ubiquitous—and to the uninitiated, mysterious—soybean.

SUBSTITUTIONS, PLEASE

For those who must restrict their intake of dairy foods, eggs, and wheat products, getting enough protein will still be no problem, because of the variety of grains, nuts and legumes to choose from. For added protein and calcium, you can eat fish products rich in both (for calcium, this includes those with bones—sardines, canned salmon—and shellfish). Fish stock made from bones will also add calcium.

Additional sources of calcium (adult RDA 800 milligrams) are:

tofu: 4-ounce serving, about 140 milligrams
miso: 1 tablespoon, about 50 milligrams
soy flour, defatted: 1 cup, about 360 milligrams
almonds: ½ cup, 155 milligrams
peanuts: 1 cup, 104 milligrams
tahini (sesame paste): ¼ cup, 40 milligrams
greens (beets, collards, kale): 1 cup, about 200 milligrams

NINE

SOY PRODUCTS AND HOW TO USE THEM

If you've already decided you like the taste of tofu (and there are many who claim it hasn't one), this chapter will have little to convince you of. But for most of us, the soybean is not naturally part of our diet, and an introduction—with personal biases thrown in—is in order. Its merits are many, so first let's talk about its drawbacks.

It's very inconvenient to cook. The soybean is a tough customer that vies favorably with small pebbles. If you're going to boil it, you almost have to resign yourself to spending several days hanging around the kitchen.

I don't like cooked soybeans per se, much as I enjoy various soy products. To me, they have a slightly bitter taste, besides taking forever to cook. Macrobiotics teachers like Muramoto also say the unadulterated soybean is hard to digest. And yet it offers the allure of that good complete protein.

The solution that Oriental peoples from Japan to Indonesia have traditionally used is to "process" the beans in a natural way, by cooking and pressing, treating them with salt and aging, or fermentation. Chief among these products are the scintillating tamari soy or shoyu sauce that serves as a salt substitute and so much more; the various kinds of miso, the fermented food that provides protein, vitamins, vital flora for the intestines, and the basic substitute for meat flavor in soups and other dishes; tofu, the bean curd that is a substitute for cheese and meat; and tempeh, an Indonesian specialty that is a substitute for ground meat because of its texture.

Our own culture has given us soy flour, soy grits and soy milk, plus a world of pre-packaged soy mixtures.

WHAT ARE THEY?

The first product that made its way to the West was the sauce we call soy. In health food stores it appears as *tamari, shoyu* and *lima soy sauce*. The reason for this somewhat schizophrenic nomenclature is that early makers of good-quality fermented soy sauce were trying to differentiate it from the more cheaply made commercial "soy sauce" found in grocery stores or sometimes in Chinese restaurants. This soy sauce is produced artificially by adding alcohol, corn syrup, salt and coloring to soy meal.

Naturally fermented soy sauce, whatever name it goes by, is the product used in macrobiotic cooking. It is most commonly called tamari. Tamari is made from naturally fermented soybeans to which salt, water and sometimes grains have been added. If you have a wheat allergy, you may want to inquire whether your tamari was made with wheat, although it is also possible that after undergoing the fermentation process the wheat will not have much effect anyway. Tamari is rich in vitamins and minerals, and contains easily digested vegetable protein.

People who have been told to cut down on their sodium intake sometimes protest that they cannot use the fermented soy products, like tamari, because they are too salty. If you are on a low-salt diet, you may want to ask for advice on how the salt-bearing soy products compare with regular salt or with the amount of sodium contained in meat. You might also look for low-sodium soy sauces now on the market. Check the labels for fermentation information.

The Nutrition Almanac (McGraw-Hill Book Co.; 1973) puts the sodium content of a teaspoon of salt at 2,132 mg, and a cup of beef bouillon at 782 mg; a cup of miso stock, made with one teaspoon of miso, contains about 850 mg of sodium. And while a pound of steak contains 343 mg of sodium, tofu is a low-sodium dieter's dream, at only 30 mg a pound! (The suggested RDA for sodium is 1,100–3,300 mg, or one-half to 1½ teaspoons of salt daily. Americans average up to nine times that much daily.)

As Oriental cuisines have become more widely known in this country, *tofu* has become probably second in popularity to tamari. It is the mild bean curd produced when soybeans are soaked and cooked and the liquid, or "soy milk," is drained off. The "milk" is then curdled and put out to set into curds and whey. The curds are then set in boxes or pans and pressed under a weighted lid for a period of half an hour or more. The result is a tofu cake, which, if made commercially, may weigh forty or fifty pounds. This will be cut into smaller cakes, usually about a pound in weight, which are sold in tofu shops, health food stores, and even supermarkets. A brand that is widely carried is Nasoya. Many health food stores carry good locally made tofu, and this is also fine. Tofu should be kept in enough water to cover in a sealed or tightly covered container in the refrigerator. The water should be changed every day or so.

Next in familiarity in Western cuisine is the soy paste called *miso*. A fermented product made from a mash of soybeans—sometimes with other grains mixed in—sea salt and water, the miso is aged for up to several years. Because it is a fermented product, it supplements the body's natural supply of "friendly" intestinal bacteria necessary for good digestion, and it is a source of vitamin B_{12}.

Three kinds of miso are generally recognized: *hacho, mugi*

Did You Know? Crumbled and sautéed, tempeh provides the meaty texture you may be craving in chili or spaghetti sauce, while miso and tamari go into stocks, soups and sauces as a stand-in for meat broths or concentrates.

and *kome*. *Hacho* is made only of soybeans and is strongest, aging as much as three years. *Mugi*, made of soybeans and barley, is milder, aging about eighteen months. *Kome*, made of soybeans and rice, is mildest; it ages only six months. The latter two are most commonly used in this country. (Miso, being a fermented food, keeps almost indefinitely. Some people don't even refrigerate it, but I do, because refrigeration seems to keep it from drying out in the climate of our centrally heated homes.) Again, if you are experiencing difficulty finding the product, it may help to have a manufacturer's name. Erewhon is one health food brand that produces miso. Westbrae is another; Westbrae's White Miso is used in some of the fancier macrobiotic dishes. Erewhon's *mugi* miso is a good everyday miso.

Tempeh, a fermented soy food, is the most recent entry on the American food scene. A staple of Indonesian cooking, tempeh is made by soaking, hulling and boiling the beans, then drying them and mixing in a bit of "starter," as is done for yogurt. The tempeh is then left to ferment for a day or so. The fermenting agent is a mold called *rhizopus*. The finished tempeh, which sometimes includes grains as well as beans, has a texture somewhat like ground meat or nut meats. According to William Shurtleff and Akiko Aoyagi in *The Book of Tofu* (Ballantine Books; 1975), tempeh is the world's richest known vegetable source of vitamin B_{12}. It is available in some health food stores; if you need a producer's name, The

Tempeh Works in Greenline, Massachusetts, and Cricklewood Soy Foods in Mertztown, Pennsylvania, are two. Tempeh keeps in the refrigerator for up to a week and can often be bought frozen.

Tofu, miso, tamari and tempeh are the great animal-food substitutes for those in need of them. Crumbled and sautéed, tempeh provides the meaty texture you may be craving in chili or spaghetti sauce, with a pleasant nutty flavor. Mashed tofu mixes with or replaces ricotta, cottage cheese and even egg in many recipes. Miso is the key ingredient for stocks and soups where a hearty flavor is wanted. Tamari goes everywhere—in sauces, stocks and basting liquids. As a companion to miso or without it, tamari serves as a good stand-in for meat broths, bouillon cubes or meat concentrates.

Other soy products that have been popular among vegetarians in this country are soy flour and soy milk. Soy flour can be used instead of regular flour in many recipes, but it imparts a stronger flavor in delicate dishes, and it does not contain the gluten needed to make bread rise. It is in fact one of the three "magic" ingredients in Cornell University's famous and delicious bread.

Soy milk can be prepared by soaking and hulling the beans, then grinding or processing them, using one part beans to three parts water if you are grinding them in a blender. They are then strained and the fluid is simmered about half an hour, stirring to prevent scorching. While the milk is still warm, a little barley malt or honey may be added (except if the milk is to be fed to young infants), and a little salt. It should be refrigerated. Soy milk has proved useful chiefly to people who are allergic to dairy foods, especially cow's milk. For adults, it is probably simpler just to substitute other drinks.

The soy milk must be boiled, by the way, because of antidigestive elements contained in raw soybeans. These substances, called soybean trypsin inhibitors, prevent the pancreatic enzyme trypsin from functioning to digest the bean and make full use of its nutrients. It is for this reason that all soy foods must be cooked, fermented, or otherwise prepared to make them digestible. Even soy sprouts are never eaten raw; they are steamed or boiled for five minutes, or lightly sautéed. It is also for this reason that cooked soybeans are not recommended in traditional macrobiotic cuisine; because they are so resistant to cooking, and because thorough cooking of the whole bean is necessary to assure destruction of the trypsin inhibitors, the fermented or curdled soy foods are preferred.

Other soy products available in health food stores, including textured soy proteins and a wide range of "instant" soy burger mixes, usually represent a degree of processing that makes them less preferable nutritionally—defatted soy flour and grits, for instance, are processed with solvents to remove the fats, and textured soy proteins are made of defatted soy flour further processed under high heat and pressure.

One other Japanese soy product is worth mentioning, since it is becoming available in some places. Called *natto*, it is made from whole soybeans, steamed and fermented with the use of a natto starter. The natto beans, like *hacho* miso, have a strong flavor, and not everyone will like them. They can be stored like miso, and are used on rice or noodles or in sautéed vegetables or soups.

WHEN TO USE THEM

For starters, try incorporating tofu and miso into your diet in a few places. The recipes for Stages Two and Three, some of which are mentioned in this section, will give you some ideas. Tamari has probably already found its way into all of our kitchens, as an occasional condiment, and in any case can be used in lieu of salt in all but the more delicate recipes.

Start with miso by adding a little to your soups. The best way is to dissolve the miso—up to a tablespoon at first—in a bit of the soup, and add to the pot near the end of cooking. Some tamari can be added as well. This works well with any of the heartier homemade soups, including pea, lentil and minestrone.

Simple Miso Soup is a good starter for a meal, or a very simple meal in itself if you are feeling a bit under the weather. It introduces two flavors quite unfamiliar to Westerners: the miso and one of the seaweeds. The soup is highly nutritious, low in calories, and very digestible. In time, its bland, mildly salty taste with a slight bitter edge will seem like an old friend; if it tastes strange at first, just try it again every once in a while.

Note that sometimes the miso curdles and doesn't blend evenly into the broth. This is probably because the liquid was a trifle too hot, but curdling doesn't affect the flavor or nutritional value of the miso.

Tofu goes well in stir-fry in lieu of meat, or in addition to fish or chicken. It can also be used to replace eggs and cheese in a number of recipes—use it to replace one or more eggs in Egg and Tofu Salad, or some cheese in Ratatouille Tofu Lasagne, or some eggs and cheese in Vegetable Quiche with Tofu. Or just eat Broiled Tofu in lieu of meat. Tofu is a cooked product when you buy it, but additional cooking makes it even more digestible. You may want to steam and cool it, for instance, before adding it to egg salad or cutting it up to put in salad.

As for tempeh, it is a great meat substitute in Meatless Moussaka, Vegetarian Chili, and Tempeh Loaf (delicious with Mushroom Gravy).

Once you get acquainted with these soy delicacies, many ways of substituting them in your own favorite recipes will occur to you. You may also find yourself making more use of a few other Oriental staples.

OTHER EXOTIC STAPLES

Seaweeds are discussed in detail in Stage Three, but you can start now by buying the handsome reddish purple *dulse* and the all-purpose dark green *wakame* (WAH-kah-may), both good in soups. Simply crumble them into minestrone or miso, or let them soak for a few minutes in cool water and them chop them and add to strong-flavored vegetables like spinach, kale or escarole while cooking. The seaweeds are rich in minerals and vitamins. If grain or bean dishes are hard to digest, try breaking a small piece of *kombu* into the cooking water.

Gomasio, an important macrobiotic condiment, is also delicious. It can be bought at some health food stores, or easily prepared if you have a mortar and pestle. It is made of sesame seeds, available at health food stores in bulk, and sea salt, and is made by roasting the seeds with sea salt.

Sesame seeds are an important ingredient in their own right. Roast them lightly in a skillet until they pop (be sure to rinse them first), and add to salads, baked goods, granola, soups, stir-fry—just about any dish. They are high in calcium and contain protein and vitamin E. They should be stored in the refrigerator.

Fresh ginger is another good Oriental ingredient. Add it to any dish that wants a little spice; try it in stir-fry. It can be chopped or grated, leaving the skin on if you wash it. The grated ginger can also be squeezed to make juice. Store in the open air, where it will tend to dry out instead of molding, as it does in the refrigerator. If the open end does mold, just slice it off and discard. Ginger is known in the Orient as a great blood purifier and as an aid to digestion.

If you can find dried shiitake (shuh-TAH-kay) mushrooms, you'll find they're good for Mushroom Gravy. More about the shiitake in Stage Three.

BEAN SPROUTS

Bean sprouts are hardly exotic for use today, available as they are in the fresh produce aisle of many grocery stores, along with alfalfa sprouts. The fat whitish sprouts most commonly available are mung bean sprouts, and are used widely in Oriental cooking, but you can sprout and use virtually any bean at home.

The reason I haven't really talked about sprouts is that they take keeping track of. They spoil quickly, in the refrigerator or the sprouter. Packages of them are bulky, and can be hard to use up unless you eat a lot of sprouts. And if you are sprouting them in a jar at home, you must remember to change the water daily, or almost. As one who has trouble remembering to water the plants, I find this tough. But if you are heading toward an all-vegetable diet, or if you just love the crunch of the protein-rich little seedlings, you should definitely make sprouts a must on your list of staples. And if you're good at remembering to water the plants, by all means grow your own.

Sprouting jars are now available at many stores where cookware is sold, and also at health food stores. You can make your own with any good-sized wide-mouthed jar, a piece of clean loose-woven cloth like cheesecloth (no dyes, please) and a rubber band. Rinse and drain ½ cup beans. Put in a jar with 2 cups warm water and let stand overnight. Drain off water; rinse thoroughly in cold water. Cover the jar mouth with the cloth and fasten with a rubber band. Set the jar, mouth down, at a tilt in a bowl in a dark cupboard. The sprouts should be ready in about three days. Store in the refrigerator for up to a week.

If your beans get moldy while sprouting, try rinsing them more often—two or three times a day—and be sure to drain thoroughly. If you are sprouting soybeans, the sprouts must be cooked for two or three minutes to destroy the enzyme inhibitor inherent in the soybean. Soybeans may take longer to sprout—up to five days; the sprouts contain fewer calories than any other known protein food. Soybean sprouts also develop vitamin C, which the dry bean lacks, and increase in B vitamins during sprouting.

With your regular staples and the addition of some new grains, beans and soy products, you are ready to be the "compleat" vegetarian, if you like. Go at your own pace. If you're ready to start cooking, the Stage Two recipes are waiting for you. Or, if your own pace right now includes some stumbling blocks—old habits or your own household—just keep reading.

TEN

LIVING WITH BOLOGNA LOVERS

As we progress at home with new and exciting forays into unfamiliar cuisines, any resistance we felt to them naturally diminishes. New recipes are tested and proved tasty and reasonably safe for family and even guests.

At the same time, there may be resistance on the home front, and if there is, dual menus may be a temporary course of least resistance. The idea of a dual menu—one meal for the meat lovers and something else for the vegetarians—grew of necessity in our kitchen as I began experimenting with vegetarian foods. My husband would eat many things, but he drew the line at tofu, and he wasn't wild about lentils. Besides, he *liked* meat, and while he was a good sport about my vegetarian odyssey, it wasn't his idea, after all. At this point, I discovered the Lentil Burger Principle.

The Lentil Burger Principle is that it's not too much trouble to cook separate dishes now and then, especially if you eat the same foods the rest of the time; sometimes you eat leftovers so there are days off for the chef; the meat eaters help; the centerpiece of the meal is the only part that's differ-

122

ent—he eats hamburger, I eat lentil burger, we both eat salad and fresh corn.

A week of meals might go like this:

- Sunday—I have time to cook, so there's meatless lasagne and we eat it with a simple salad, and maybe a glass of wine. If it's summer there's lettuce from the garden.
- Monday—a hectic day at work and I don't want to bother cooking. Thank goodness for leftover lasagne. Paul picks up some Italian rolls on his way home from work.
- Tuesday—Paul feels like meat. I have some lentil burgers in the freezer, because I have learned from hard experience that you can't make them from scratch in the time it takes to fry a hamburger. I stop at the store for hamburger for Paul and get whole wheat muffins, lettuce and tomato for our burgers. (He helps by frying his while I cook mine.)
- Wednesday—we're in a hurry to get to a movie so I fix noodles milanese because they have the virtue of being very quick. Salad on the side or some steamed broccoli or zucchini, which were part of my weekly shopping trip.
- Thursday—supplies are getting low, but I can put together a Potage Bonne Femme from our staple vegetables, with toasted or grilled cheese sandwiches.
- Friday—I set a little steak out to thaw in the morning. Tonight I can make either stir-fry with brown rice (I'll call and ask Paul to put it on as I leave the office), with steak in his stir-fry and tofu in mine, or he can have steak, baked potato and steamed vegetables and I'll have baked potato, yogurt or cottage cheese and steamed vegetables.
- Saturday—We have dinner guests. I get scallops and flounder from the fish store, to be poached in wine, and we eat them over rice with steamed vegetables, with ice cream and cooked apples for dessert.

By now I know what foods we both like and how often I have the time and patience for complicated cooking. I'm lucky also to have a dinner partner who isn't a fussy eater. If your household includes finicky eaters, try to be patient and don't be defensive. Some foods are a problem to some people —beets, for instance, or strong-flavored greens. Don't insist on the "harder" foods, but don't be a doormat either. Let the problem eaters fend for themselves as much as possible.

THE SINGLE DINER

Given our society's changing structure, a lot of people today are saying, "But what about the person who lives alone?" It is all very well to talk about buying smaller portions, but a pepper is after all a pepper. Fortunately, a great many things, peppers included, keep for a long time in a relatively good condition. This is especially true of the ingredients we have established as staples.

The trick to having the ingredients you want on hand without wasting food by spoilage is to subdivide supplies mentally into things that will spoil and things that won't. If you have the staples (things that won't spoil) on hand, you know you can always make spaghetti and clam sauce, or tuna casserole, or stir-fried vegetables over rice, with what you have in the house.

With the added staples in Stage Two, much the same thing is true. Miso keeps practically forever, as do dried seaweed and dried mushrooms. With staple vegetables and grains on hand, you can have a hearty or light miso soup any time, plus some kind of healthy entrée.

What don't keep well are certain other vegetarian ingredients, notably tofu and tempeh. Tofu lasts really only days, and this can be a nuisance because tofu is usually sold in pound portions, and a pound of tofu goes a long way. If you can find a store that sells locally made tofu, you may be able to buy smaller quantities.

In any case, plan when you buy, so that you don't get tofu

and tempeh at the same time. Use some of the soy product right away, and if there's too much to eat within four or five days, cook it into something that can be frozen—lasagne for the tofu, and vegetarian chili or moussaka for the tempeh. The quality of the soy products, like most other things, is altered by freezing, and the texture degenerates somewhat, as does the total nutritional value. But this is true of other frozen foods as well, and the frozen cooked soy dishes are perfectly palatable. Also, the soy products when cooked will keep for up to a week if properly refrigerated. They actually improve in taste with sitting.

One woman I knew who was studying macrobiotics became fixated on the size of the daikon radishes. They were pretty big, and she was sure she couldn't possibly use up even *one*. I suggested she try splitting one with another cook who didn't need a whole one; it is one solution. If you know other people who are cooking in small quantities—share the ingredients that come in unwieldy amounts. On the other hand, the radish is a root vegetable, and like a carrot will keep for weeks, if not months—though, to be sure, the freshest vegetable is the most nutritious.

In planning your cooking so as not to overstock your larder, you will have to experiment at first. Maybe you'll use a lot of dried split peas and lentils. These keep for months. But if you find they don't get used up, next time buy only one or the other. Likewise millet, bulgur and kasha—you may want to have only one on hand at a time. After finishing one, plan on recipes that will use up another. This could include adapting recipes that call for some other grain, or mixing grains that take about the same amount of time to cook—millet and rice, or kasha and bulgur, or barley with any of these. Or add the shorter cooking grain to the longer when the latter is partly done.

Another problem of the single diner is that it can frankly be a drag to cook and eat alone, so there will be times when you'll want to eat out. When I lived by myself, I made a point of taking myself out to dinner once a week—usually after work during the week—to give myself a break from coming home from the office to fix dinner and create dirty dishes. It wasn't necessarily fancy, but I did it once a week. I also fasted for all or most of a day once a week, usually on a weekend, when I could arrange to be without distractions and frustrations. Which brings us to the subject of . . .

FEASTING AND FASTING

Taking a leaf from the peoples of the Bible, consider the philosophy of the fatted calf: that is to say, there are those foods that you may still eat occasionally, although it does not serve you well to eat them often. These are the foods you may want to keep as part of your diet, to be eaten only on very special occasions.

The flip side of feasting is fasting, whatever form it takes. It too was no stranger to people of the Bible, who customarily ate very simply and sometimes not at all. You define the limits of your own form of fasting. It may be just eating very simply for a twenty-four-hour period, or eating fewer meals during that period, or consuming only liquids. Whatever it is, it should not be haphazard. Most experts recommend drinking liquids during a fast period. An extended fast should be undertaken only with adequate supervision, but a fast of a day's duration, consuming only liquids, is a way of letting the body rest, and benefits the digestive organs. People who fast once a week for a day often make it a juice fast, or consume only water and a simple soup. An energy-rich "tea" for fasting is made of spring water brought to a boil, with ½ tablespoon blackstrap unsulfured molasses per cup and the juice of ½ lemon mixed in, to be sipped at intervals during the fast day for nutrition (the molasses is rich in iron and B vitamins, the lemon in vitamin C).

The concepts of feasting and fasting were universally

known in traditional cultures, though we tend to assume that they didn't eat the fatted calf very often for economic reasons, and that they fasted for arcane religious reasons. Mankind was not meant to do either in excess. Naboru Muramoto, in *Healing Ourselves*, expresses the same idea with regard to alcohol: "This is good in its own time. The trouble is, people usually take it because they have a problem. Worse, they take it to forget. Where there is a gathering to celebrate some great event, one drinks to *remember* that event . . . having a small glass or even two. A happy occasion nullifies the bad effects of alcohol. Ask yourself how many occasions are like that."

Your idea of a feast will vary with your degree of vegetarianism. This year it might be beef and wine; next year, it might be fish and herb tea.

THE VEGETARIAN DINNER GUEST

By now your friends are all aware that you eschew meat, and it's no problem because they either like fish and pasta, or they don't care if you bring your own food.

For people who don't know you as well, you might ask if you can bring a dish. If they say no, explain why you are offering to do so. If they don't say they were actually planning a fish dinner anyway, offer again, saying that you frequently bring a nonmeat entrée for yourself, and would that be all right? If this is out of the question, and you can't bring yourself to do it, we are probably talking about the boss or your Great-aunt Minerva. Strategies here include eating the meat or disposing of it when no one is looking.

MENU PLANNING

Recipes for Stage Two are intended as a bridge between a diet that includes flesh foods and a diet that is centered on grains and vegetables. The recipes are an eclectic mix from various cuisines, but of course they reflect my preferences—that's why you'll find a preponderance of mushrooms, carrots, celery, and brown rice, for instance. Be sure to experiment freely with the grains and vegetables to include your own favorites, too.

Many of the recipes in Stage Two represent minor adaptations of techniques and recipes from Stage One. The soups especially can travel with us from Stage One right into Stage Three, since we started by making them without any meat-based stocks, except for the chicken soups. And the gradual vegetarian may want to carry some other foods over from one stage to the next, especially for special occasions.

Thus while a Stage One vegetarian might eat red meat occasionally, a Stage Two vegetarian might eat poultry occasionally, and a Stage Three vegetarian might eat dairy foods sometimes. It is worth remembering, again, that even strict macrobiotic diets allow fish occasionally. So unless you have personal reasons for wishing to eat only plant food, you can keep on eating fish regularly, at least in Stage Two.

Some other things to keep in mind:

■ Try to limit the use of dairy food so that it is the center-piece of no more than one meal a day. Otherwise you may be eating too much fat. This means that if you're having lasagne for dinner, you should be eating something other than cheese sandwiches for lunch.

■ Have one "feast" a week—one meal where the family is present and has time to relax and enjoy. Dinner needn't be a seven-course meal, but should be something every-one likes. Lasagne, shish-kebabs, stir-fry, chili, tacos, Pasta Primavera and fish are some popular choices. The meal can include salad, bread, wine and/or dessert with little extra trouble.

▪ Try to fix at least one meal a week where soy products or grains are the centerpiece.

▪ Don't neglect your fresh vegetables, raw or cooked.

▪ Do make use of your staples during midweek, and cook— even freeze—large batches of food in advance, especially if all the adults in the family work.

▪ If any family members express an interest, try to encourage involvement in the menu-planning process. Solicit requests for favorites before the week's shopping.

▪ Keep your sense of humor.

ELEVEN

BEHAVIOR MODIFICATION

At this point in our diets, we are capable of quitting meats altogether. That is, we know enough about the nutritional alternatives and the delicious variety of alternatives.

We also know about the pitfalls—dinner with Aunt Minnie, lunch at McDonald's, breakfast on the run. And then there's backsliding, which is fine if it's what we want to do. But what if it isn't?

When it came to changing my diet, I found my attitudes had been shaped by my experience quitting smoking. It took a number of tries over a period of years, but I just kept doing the best I could. It was basically a process of behavior modification. The same thing works for food. So if things aren't going the way you want them to, here are a few thoughts:

- Be conscious of what you're doing. Random, chaotic and thoughtless eating—following the whim of a moment, or letting outside pressures dictate—is the enemy of a good diet. Set goals and try to be aware of whether they are working. If not, try to know why not. And as a psychologist I knew once said, "Do wrong or feel guilty, but don't do both—it's too much trouble."

■ Continue to analyze likes and dislikes, remembering that our "needs" in food often have an emotional and cultural basis, but that this does not make them any less valid. Be patient with the things that may taste strange or sour or bitter at first—miso and seaweed were difficult for me— trying them in small quantities or in a dish that masks their flavor if necessary. Keep experimenting.

■ Think grains and legumes as the center of the meal. It's all right for dairy foods to occupy an important place too, but make a conscious effort to limit them, remembering that they are relatively high in fat and are mucus-forming. Eat fish at least once a week, unless it conflicts with your principles.

■ If a "sweet tooth" is the problem, read *Sugar Blues* by William Dufty, and follow up on his suggestion: read the label of every food product in the house and throw out everything that contains sugar (this includes corn syrup and all sweeteners), but for the time being keep using honey, molasses and barley malt.

■ Cut down extreme foods. This means letting go of any habit that seems to have more control of you than you do of it, and cutting down on others. For instance, salt in certain quantities is vital to health, but most of us eat it thoughtlessly and in greater quantities than we need. For most of us, cutting down is a matter of simply paying attention. But if you compulsively indulge in salty snacks, then something is definitely out of balance, and this habit is in control. Treat it as an addiction of sorts, and actively weed it out. The same goes for chocolate, sugar, caffeine, alcohol and drugs of all kinds, from medication to tobacco.

Chocolate and cola lovers should be reminded that their favorite foods are not by any means harmless, despite the fact that we feed them to children as treats. Chocolate candy not only contains high levels of sugar and caffeine, but also fatty acids deleterious to our digestive and circulatory systems.

Colas frequently contain caffeine and of course either sugar or artificial sweeteners.

You *can* quit these habits. And quitting them and improving your diet are symbiotic. Also, quitting any one of them makes it easier to quit the others, because they aggravate each other. Tobacco is hardest because it is physically addictive, and unlike foods, does not have an easy natural substitute.

To begin quitting a habit, first analyze the situations in which it asserts itself. Is it a defense? A reward? A form of revenge against ourselves or the world? Try to identify the source of the self-destructive behavior, the reason why it "pays." If it is a reward—say, for finishing a job—find a substitute: eat an apple or a low-fat, high-fiber cracker instead of pie, or go for a little walk instead of smoking a cigarette. If the habit is a defense or some form of self-sabotage, try to find a more appropriate channel for resolving the problem.

The second step in quitting a habit is to remind yourself of all the good reasons for quitting. Read everything you can about why it is a bad habit and how it undermines your health, and then simply remind yourself that the extreme foods run counter to the body's process of balancing itself through better diet.

The third thing to do, as you continue to reinforce quitting or cutting down, is not to waste any energy feeling guilty if you backslide. The best way to quit a habit is to take a leaf from the book of the champion quitters, Alcoholics Anonymous, and do it one day at a time.

And remember, the best reason for quitting the extreme foods is not that they might prove carcinogenic years from now—that is not an *immediate* enough reason—but that they are holding you back from better health and better communication with your body *right now*, today and tomorrow.

TAKE YOUR TIME

As you work on changing your eating habits, be sure to take your time when shopping or ordering food or refreshments in a restaurant or bar. Don't let yourself be stampeded into ordering an alcoholic beverage or a rich entrée or dessert if that's not what you want. If you rush, you will succumb to old habits. Give yourself time to remember why some foods aren't good for you; how you felt the last time you ate them; and what might be a reasonable substitute.

If you know what restaurant or what kind of restaurant you are going to, make up a tentative menu for yourself before you actually get there. If you know you must go to a bar or a social function where cocktails will be served, set your strategy: plain seltzer water or club soda with a twist, or one beer, glass of wine or whisky and water followed by plain soda, or whatever. If you are going to a party where it would not be impolite to bring your own, take along plain soda or Perrier, fruit juice or iced herb tea. Do the same with food when possible. And at parties, receptions and the like, scan the hors d'oeuvres until you find the platters of raw vegetables, stuffed eggs and cheese and crackers, and stick with them.

In an era when so many social structures are breaking down, food remains one of the few things people can agree on and share, and this makes quitting old habits even scarier. To refuse to share food is something we have been programmed for centuries to regard as a deeply hostile act. And food is also one of the few remnants of ethnic culture that we can share with family and friends.

This is to say, once more, that no one should feel discouraged if changing eating and drinking habits comes hard. If it comes easy, we may count ourselves lucky indeed.

THE
GRADUAL
VEGETARIAN

STAGE THREE

TWELVE

The Various Vegetarians

A friend of mine had been suffering from various ailments including a persistent irritation of the eyes. She rubbed them all the time, and she said it felt like sandpaper on the inside of her lids. Her job as an editor depended on her eyes, and nothing conventional had helped. She was desperate for relief.

She went to see a macrobiotics specialist who had just opened a business near her home. He and his wife taught macrobiotic cooking as a way of healing.

The editor didn't tell him specifically what was wrong, but as he examined her he peered into her eyes, turning down her eyelids.

"You've been eating a lot of chicken," he remarked.

It was true, but how did he know? He pointed out the irritation of the eyelids, which she hadn't mentioned. "That's from eating too much poultry," he said.

She was somewhat astonished. But there was more. She had been diagnosed by a gynecologist as having endometriosis, for which the doctor said the only remedy might be surgery. Pregnancy, the doctor added, sometimes helped.

But she had already been trying to get pregnant, with no success.

The macrobiotics specialists gave her a little lecture on the stress to internal organs caused by the typical American diet. What did she have to lose? She professed doubts about her ability to live on seaweed and brown rice. Every little bit would help, they told her. She took classes and incorporated some of their philosophy into her diet. Today her eyes are better and she is the proud mother of a little boy. The endometriosis is gone.

Was it coincidence? Psychology? Natural healing? She says she doesn't know. But whatever it was, it worked.

Among stricter vegetarian diets are some that people embark on for health reasons. Macrobiotics in its strictest form is one of them. The trouble with all of these diets, from the casual observer's viewpoint, is the lack of conventional scientific proof of their claims. Like my friend, we are left wondering what works, and why. Should we post a sign that says, "Beware—the fringe!"?

Stage Three is devoted to examining some of the diets that lie beyond the conventional lacto-ovo-vegetarian middle of the road. It attempts to identify them, sort them out, and introduce cooking ideas for two of them. It is worth noting at this point that not everyone will stay on a strict vegetarian diet, but that we may try them for a time and return to them as needed. We can certainly find useful ideas for healthier cooking here, to incorporate into whatever diet we decide on. The thing to remember, once again, is not to mix up eating styles chaotically. Moderation in all things is a good motto.

One of the diets we'll examine is macrobiotics, introducing some unfamiliar ingredients including seaweeds and various new condiments. The other is natural hygiene, an American philosophy based on eating simply prepared fruits and vegetables. We'll be looking at what it's like to do without most animal foods, including dairy products.

I was pleasantly surprised when I began trying the Stage

Three diets, especially macrobiotics. I approached it warily. On the first spoonful of my teacher's soup, I would think, "Too bland." But by the third spoonful, the delicate flavors would get past the years of overseasoned foods that had jaded my palate, and I would murmur with satisfaction, "Delicious."

The Stage Three diets represent a much larger step away from what we grew up with, but again, remember: You don't have to do it all at once. Or forever. As the teacher said, every little bit helps.

A QUESTION OF BALANCES

One of the mysteries of human existence is how cultures that technically knew nothing about nutrition have instinctively combined foods properly to obtain all the necessary nutrients for a balanced diet. It took us until the twentieth century to identify amino acids and to decide that not all foods contain complete proteins. Meanwhile, what were uneducated people in traditional cultures doing? They were routinely eating combinations of grains, legumes and nuts in a way that provided complete protein.

At any stage in our diet, we can learn to pay attention to what our bodies and traditional cultures have to tell us. What is appropriate at one stage may not be appropriate at another. Let us pause and consider where our exploration of the beginning stages of vegetarianism may have brought us. What new habits have we developed? Are they balanced or could they, too, be harmful? For instance, if we have eaten meat and other animal fats heavily over the years, one reaction to quitting them may be a craving for fats, which could translate into using cooking oil, butter or dairy foods too frequently.

So an increase in the amount of oils and other non-meat fats may be a sign of changing habits that we may understand and accept, giving ourselves some leeway. This is all right as long as we don't overdo it, keeping in mind that an excess of fats of any kind will eventually clog the system. And we should keep in mind that this, like meat-eating, may be a transition to another diet—it does not have to be a permanent way of life.

This is just one of the body's instinctive balancing acts. Many nutritional balances are built into traditional diets. Take the family of recipes that have come to us from southern Italy and elsewhere along the Mediterranean. Tomatoes, according to Naboru Muramoto, help eliminate excess stored animal protein from the body. So it is perhaps not surprising that we instinctively turn to many tomato-rich Mediterranean dishes as the central dishes in our diet when we first quit eating meats—dishes like lasagne, ravioli, ratatouille, even pizza.

But it is also interesting to note several other key ingredients of these dishes. First, they typically are made with olive oil, one of the heavier plant oils, which may make them especially appealing to someone whose diet contains less animal fat than before. Second, tomatoes are high in oxalic acid, which is known to combine with vital calcium, removing it from use in the body as a bone builder; but the Mediterranean tomato-based dishes almost invariably contain large amounts of cheese, a dairy food and, of course, high in calcium.

Third, while the cheese is relatively high in fat and cholesterol—unless it's a low-fat cheese like cottage cheese—these dishes also are typically made with garlic. Garlic has been revered in cultures from Egypt to India and from Rome to Ireland as a healing plant that was supposed to impart strength to workers and passion to lovers, cure respiratory ailments, aid digestion and combat internal parasites. Modern studies reported in *Lancet*, the British medical journal (Dec. 29, 1973), showed garlic was effective in lowering cholesterol levels in humans, and reducing blood fat and blood sugar levels in laboratory animals. Onions were also part of the latter study. The studies likewise suggested these two related vegetables would prove effective against diabetes.

This does not mean that we have license to go out and make pizza a mainstay of our diet. But in trying to surmise what our bodies and traditional diets may tell us about eating properly, we might conclude that if we are craving dishes rich in tomatoes and garlic, and eating them frequently, our bodies may still be dealing with an overload of animal protein, stored over years of eating far more of it than we needed. And we also may be dealing with an overload of sugar, which our bodies are striving to balance.

TRY, TRY AGAIN

As our habits change, it is also important to keep an open mind about foods we always thought we didn't like. Foods that formerly had no place in our lives may suddenly become quite delicious. We should keep trying the foods that are especially healthy, even if at first not all of them are favorites.

In some of our new foods, we will find nutritional substitutes for old standbys. We discover, for instance, that sesame seeds and some of the seaweeds are high in calcium. The sesame seeds can enter our diets as sesame oil, tahini (sesame paste), sesame butter, gomasio or whole roasted seeds—all pleasant tasting. The seaweeds, while we may be less sure of them, can be added unobtrusively at first. Together these new foods mean that we can let go of some of our old sources of a vital nutrient like calcium without feeling panicky.

And it is important to remember that today's favorite may be tomorrow's extreme food. Today, bananas may be especially attractive, and perhaps it's because their high potassium content is helping us balance a high level of sodium within our bodies.

But as we eat less salt, less meat and less of other sodium-rich foods, the time may come when bananas are not a really useful food for us anymore, but are too extreme, being a tropical food and not native to our predominantly temperate climate. On the other hand, for someone living in the desert or subtropical parts of the country, a diet rich in hot-weather and even tropical fruits and vegetables might be perfectly appropriate.

THE ELUSIVE IDEAL DIET

There are widely divergent opinions among vegetarians about what constitutes the ideal diet, and each school is convinced that its own way is best. This can be quite confusing to anyone who is trying to approach the subject with an open mind and make a sensible decision about his or her own diet. And there are other confusing messages coming from other sources, ranging from the government to specific industries; the latter may or may not identify themselves as such.

Our health is so important to us, and ill health so expensive, that nutrition naturally becomes an emotional issue. Whom can you trust?

VARIOUS VEGETARIANS

Beyond the lacto-ovo-vegetarians there are several major philosophies about what is best to eat if one is not going to eat a traditional meat-centered diet.

There is the macrobiotic approach, which was derived from a traditional Japanese diet and introduced to the West by George Ohsawa and his followers. It emphasizes cooked vegetables and grains and soy foods, and de-emphasizes fruits and raw vegetables, especially tropical ones.

There is a vegetarian approach derived from Hindu cooking. Like the macrobiotic system, it holds that certain foods are healing for certain conditions, as it disallows pollutants like drugs, refined sugars, alcohol, caffeine and tobacco. But it places more emphasis on raw foods and fruits, including tropical fruits.

In this country a philosophy has developed that goes one step further, and is perhaps best represented by the writings of Dr. Herbert M. Shelton of San Antonio, Texas. Shelton, a self-styled "hygienist," holds that raw fruit and vegetables are the ideal human food.

There are also fruitarians, who hold that it is unethical to eat anything that causes the destruction of any living organism or otherwise interrupts the ongoing process of life on the planet, be it animal or plant. For them, only fruits of plants—not roots, or leaves, or even seeds and nuts, since these are life carriers—are acceptable foods.

Vegans are plant eaters who avoid all animal foods, including of course milk products, eggs and animal-based gelatin, but also the less obvious honey, since it is produced by bees. There are other degrees of vegetarianism where it is acceptable to eat animal food only if it has involved no killing: thus milk and yogurt might be all right, but eggs might not be. Cheese is unacceptable unless it is rennetless cheese, since the coagulant rennet used in cheese making is extracted from animal stomachs.

MACROBIOTICS

Macrobiotics is a dietary style with roots in a philosophy that is esoteric to the Western mind. But in practical terms it has much to offer, as perhaps the next most logical step beyond lacto-ovo-vegetarianism.

George Ohsawa (1892–1966) led the development of the macrobiotic system of diet in pre–World War II Japan. His teachings spread to the United States in the 1950s. The East-West Institute, founded in Boston in the 1960s by Michio Kushi, has been the center of macrobiotics teaching from which other East-West centers have developed in major cities of the country, including Baltimore, Chicago, Miami, New York, Philadelphia and Washington, D.C. There are also affiliates in smaller cities and in Canada and England.

Kushi defines macrobiotics as a compassionate discipline that takes the largest possible view of life (the name comes from the Greek words *macro*, large, and *bios*, life).

Philosophically, macrobiotics speaks of food as a form of packaging for the energy that sustains life. The energy, called *ki*, manifests itself in the balancing of the eternal opposite principles of Yin and Yang, which are seen, in Oriental philosophy, in all aspects of the universe. Yin and Yang are often popularly referred to as feminine and masculine principles, but for the purposes of understanding the macrobiotic diet it is more useful to know that they are also thought of in terms of expansion and contraction; cold and heat; moisture and dryness; darkness and sunlight. The macrobiotic diet attempts to regulate the flow of *ki* by balancing food intake and preparation in terms of Yin and Yang. It does this for the sake of spiritual advancement, but also in quest of good physical health.

Foods are considered more Yin or more Yang in terms of how and where they grow, and also in terms of their effects on us. Thus foods that grow rapidly—tropical fruits and to a lesser extent fruits in general—are considered aligned with the expansive principle, or Yin. Foods that grow more slowly, thrive in a colder climate or contain much nourishment in compact form are more Yang. A seed is more Yang than a fruit. Root crops—our winter vegetables—are said to be Yang. Meat and salt are Yang. Substances that are said to have an expanding, or Yin, effect on us include those that cause us to "get out of ourselves," as we like to say: drugs, alcohol, sugar and tobacco. Macrobiotics encourages a diet that is perceived as striking the ideal balance, avoiding excesses of Yang or Yin. The diet, therefore, centers on grains, with complementary dishes that are modestly Yin (some fruits, leafy greens, quick-growing vegetables) or Yang (root vegetables, beans, some salty soy foods and salt in cooking, but no salt, which is perhaps the most extremely Yang food, eaten directly).

Some interesting claims have been made for the healthy properties of a macrobiotic diet. Health articles are a regular feature of *East-West Journal*, and among them have been Leonard Jacobs's article in June 1979 about macrobiotic diet as a way of preventing and/or curing radiation sickness. More recently, Anthony Sattilaro, a Philadelphia physician, has told in *Recalled by Life* (Houghton Mifflin; 1982) the story of his self-cure, using macrobiotics, of cancer. These are just two of the more dramatic claims made for macrobiotics.

Setting these grander possible benefits aside, the macrobiotic diet is a practical step for the gradual vegetarian because it offers equivalents to some foods we are already used to, and uses many other foods—grains, legumes, vegetables and fruits—that we are eating already. It provides whole menus that are not too different from a conventional Western diet—though some of the ingredients may be unfamiliar.

Its drawbacks are that it does require some adapting in terms of taste and cooking styles, and some investment in new cooking tools. And for people on a low-sodium diet it must be approached carefully, best under expert supervision, since some of the soy foods and seaweeds are high in sodium.

Proponents of diets that emphasize more raw foods also object to the volume of cooked food, especially cooked grain, that the diet entails. They say that the cooked foods cause congestion in the intestinal tract and are nutritionally inferior.

On balance, the macrobiotic diet is one of the most important of the options available to vegetarians from a standpoint of social integration and nutrition, and as such we will examine it in more detail in the next chapter. But first, let us look at a contrasting option.

NATURAL HYGIENE

Another school of thought—possibly the major other school of thought in this country—that regards vegetarian eating as a way to health is the hygienist philosophy. Hygienists would agree with Dr. Jonathan Wright of *Prevention* magazine that human beings are essentially, digestively, the same creatures they were ten thousand years ago, and are not meant to be eating great quantities of grain or dairy food. Following the same line of thought, they say that humankind is not meant to eat great amounts of cooked food. They eschew refined foods utterly and frown on the use of cooked grains as well.

While the hygienists argue that we are, in terms of digestion, the same creatures we were before the advent of cooking fires, macrobiotics teachers like Michio Kushi believe that humankind's great growth of intelligence and development of culture was not only concurrent with, but actually a result of, unlocking the compact nutritional potential of the grain foods. That is one reason why they make cooked grains the centerpiece of every meal.

Central to the hygienists' practice of eating is the idea that digestion is more efficient if only one kind of food is eaten at a time. Herbert M. Shelton, in his *Superior Nutrition* (San Antonio; 1978), says:

> It is a matter of common experience that we tend to eat much more food when we eat two or more foods, than when we take but one at a meal . . . a variety of foods tends to induce overeating. . . . A morbid appetite, thus established [by overeating], is really just a nervous craving for stimulation. . . . Normal demands are never painful.
>
> There are other reasons why a variety of foods should not be eaten. . . . Simple meals digest better and with less tax on the digestive organs. . . . Digestion is most efficient when but one food is eaten at a time.

The hygienists' concern is focused on what happens in the digestive tract. Different types of food require different digestive secretions, and a system of "food combining" has developed accordingly. Foods that cannot be digested quickly and efficiently are considered the root of modern illness, because they remain in the digestive system too long and produce toxins.

Food villains for the hygienists are bread and cereals; overeating in general; combinations of bread and meat, bread and eggs, bread and cheese, cereals with milk or sugar, acids with starches, acids with proteins, fats with proteins; and all kinds of sweet baked goods.

Animal foods, even meat, are not necessarily excluded, but flesh foods are condemned as being deficient in minerals, vitamins and carbohydrates.

Hygienists acknowledge that few people will actually go so far as to eat only one food at a meal. Their rules of food combining offer guidance to what they consider the healthiest dietary habits. In general, foods that do not "combine" well are not taken at the same meal.

Green vegetables are at the center of the hygienist diet, because they combine well with the foods Westerners rely on most heavily: proteins and starches. Proteins are considered to include all flesh foods, dairy foods, nuts, some legumes and olives. Starches include grains, some legumes and starchy vegetables.

Fruits are considered to combine poorly with everything except other fruits and in some cases nuts or fats. Fruits are subdivided as sweet, sub-acid and acid. Sweet and acid fruits are not combined, but acid fruits may be eaten with nuts, and sweet or sub-acid fruits may be combined with yogurt or cream on occasion. In general, fruits are eaten at a "fruit meal."

WHERE DO WE GO FROM HERE?

One advantage that lacto-ovo-vegetarianism and macrobiotics offer over the more restricted diets is greater flexibility. The further we go from the conventional American diet, the more limited become our choices. This will not stop the determined fruitarian or vegan, of course, nor should it; but it may necessitate moving to an environment where the diet can be followed while still maintaining health. It will not do, for instance, to try to become a fruitarian if one is going to have to rely on canned fruit cocktail at the local diner.

We have come thus far together, through Stages One and Two. At this point, paths may well diverge, as gradual vegetarians choose their next step. Raw food or cooked? Some animal food or none? Ethical considerations, or practical, or both?

"A man of my spiritual intensity," playwright George Bernard Shaw is supposed to have remarked, "does not eat corpses." Alas, poor George! He developed pernicious anemia, for which the only known cure at the time was liver shots—which he took, much the horror of his vegetarian associates—and he lived to the age of 94.

We have come a long way, and our choices are many. Unlike Shaw, we can profit from the dietary groundwork that has already been laid.

THIRTEEN

Two Diets, One Goal

As mentioned earlier, the act of moving to a vegetarian diet seems to be inspired either by moral and ethical considerations—feeding the world's hungry, eating no food that involves killing—or by a quest for better health, be it physical or spiritual or both.

For people who are vegetarians for moral or ethical reasons, the question is primarily one of what to eat, and not of how to prepare it, as long as it is appealing. Thus someone who is primarily concerned with feeding the world's hungry might not be bothered at all by using canned tomato sauce, while someone who was seeking improved health might insist on making the tomato sauce from scratch or not use tomato sauce because it did not fit into a particular diet.

For people whose concerns are ethical, then, cooking style is less a problem than for those who are trying to change their diet for better health. At the same time, people who are planning to become stricter vegetarians for ethical reasons would be wise to consider health, too, so that when they restrict their diets they will not be forfeiting their health.

So, for both health-oriented and ethical vegetarians, we want to take a closer look at two diets that are a step beyond

lacto-ovo-vegetarianism: macrobiotics and hygienism, introduced in the last chapter. Of the health-oriented diets, these
two styles seem to me best suited for people who are adapting from more traditional Western diets, probably via lacto-
ovo-vegetarianism. While neither of them insists on a totally
vegetarian diet, at least at first, both of them *can* be totally
vegetarian.

These two diets are examined in some detail because each
involves a philosophy about how food is prepared—what is
eaten with what, and how much it is cooked—or not cooked.
These are considerations for people who are trying to adjust
their health, and for them it is important to know what the
macrobiotic meal or the practice of food combining entails.

For people who are going beyond a lacto-ovo-vegetarian
diet to become vegans, the macrobiotic diet should be studied, since non-animal sources of B_{12} (tempeh) and calcium
(seaweed, sesame seeds and bancha tea) will be needed. For
people who are primarily interested in not killing animals or
in improving the world's food supply, the wide range of recipes from lacto-ovo-vegetarianism and macrobiotics can be
used and adapted at will.

I hope that those who are contemplating going into more
restricted diets such as fruitarianism—in recent years, even
sproutarians have emerged—will be patient and do it gradually, going through one of the diets that is closer to our
present diet first. Years ago, when macrobiotics was first being publicized widely in this country, many new students
were ambitious to attain the greatest benefits of the diet immediately, and severe malnutrition resulted for some who
went on what macrobiotics teachers classify as a Number 7
diet, consisting almost exclusively of brown rice. This
overzealousness led the American Medical Association's
Council on Foods and Nutrition to issue a warning that the
macrobiotic diet was one of the most dangerous dietary regimens.

Today, no reputable macrobiotics teacher or book would

suggest that a student go directly or even quickly to a Number 7 diet from a traditional Western diet. For some of us, that is an ambition not to be entertained even in a lifetime. And Ohsawa himself is supposed to have advised his students not to undertake a brown rice diet without consulting him first.

If the diet is much better understood these days, it also comes much better equipped. In the decade since the AMA issued its warning, macrobiotics has really taken root in this country and is taught in East-West foundations all over the nation. Macrobiotic restaurants are to be found in major cities and small towns, and the health food stores that supply restaurants and individuals carry foods that were virtually unobtainable in the United States a decade ago. So, as understanding has increased of where the vitamin C, vitamin E, calcium and protein are to come from, the source foods have become abundant—the bancha tea, the seaweed, the soy products and fresh, organically grown vegetables.

In changing our dietary habits, it is also extremely important to remember that we were not all born with the same metabolism. Some people can withstand anything and come out in the pink of health.

For most of us, however, a plain brown rice or even fruitarian diet will not be advisable for many years, if ever. W. D. Kelley makes this point in his article on "The Metabolic Types" (in *One Answer to Cancer*, W. D. and Suzi Kelley, Valenkel Press; 1979). He relates how he met an Indian swami at the home of a friend and was amazed to watch the man imbibe quantities of refined sugar in water.

> Believe me, I wasted no time in getting a blood sample from him. Later, when we ran the guru's blood through our computer, I was shocked to find him in very good health. This man had four generations before him that he knew of, who were strict vegetarians never having had a bite of meat. There were probably more than four generations, but that was all he knew

of for sure. This man was as close to being a pure Metabolic Type I, a strict vegetarian, as one could ever hope to find. Most Americans do not have that type of heredity and would not fit into the strict vegetarian class.

Without going into his types too deeply—his Type I thrives on plant food, can eat up to 100 percent of it raw, and burns carbohydrates slowly, maintaining an even blood sugar level —Kelley's central thesis is that metabolism is to some extent inherited. He believes that it has been genetically determined over centuries, even millennia, by available food sources, so that people in the tropics are metabolically programmed to thrive on a high-sugar fruit diet, while people near the Arctic Circle survive successfully on a diet of virtually all animal food. America is problematical for him because it is a genetic melting pot, where he goes on to discover new metabolic types, some healthy and some not so healthy. But for most of us, his point about vegetarianism is well taken: few of our ancestors, at least recently, have observably been vegetarians, and while this may be what nature intended for us—as Jonathan Wright and Herbert Shelton would argue— it is certainly not what we have been doing recently, and it may take some undoing to get back to basics.

From this standpoint, macrobiotics (as taught by the East-West foundations in this country) and hygienism seem to be the most promising of the diets designed to return us to more wholesome foods. The macrobiotic diet is perhaps a better choice, at least at first, for those who live in the temperate and colder parts of the country; it is more in line with what our metabolism is used to if we live in those areas, with its emphasis on grains, locally grown vegetables and fruits, and cooked foods, and its avoidance of tropical fruits and vegetables.

Hygienism, on the other hand, with its emphasis on raw fruits and vegetables and its inclusion of tropical and semi-tropical plant foods, might be a workable choice for those who live in the tropical and subtropical climates. These are the climates Shelton recommends in *Food Combining Made Easy* (San Antonio; 1976), and both his Hygienic Institute and the American Natural Hygiene Society are located in the South—in Texas and Florida, respectively. The name of the controversial *Beverly Hills Diet*, with its emphasis on raw fruits, speaks for the climate in which it was conceived, and illustrates the point.

So in adjusting your diet, please keep in mind these factors: the possible needs of your own particular metabolism, which should become apparent to you if you pay attention to what you eat and how you feel; and the possible relevance of climate to diet.

The other factor to keep in mind is the social environment. East-West foundations and their affiliates are now located from Florida to Canada and from Massachusetts to California. Macrobiotics as a way of life has become relatively well entrenched in the last decade, and as a social support system you will find classes, restaurants, health food stores and like-minded individuals in many parts of the country. And while the philosophy may seem esoteric, the actual structure of the meals is not so different from what we are used to. Hygienism, while it goes back to the nineteenth century, appears less widely known. And while its language is more familiar, being purely American, its dietary demands are more stringent and are bound to be less convenient unless you live in an area where good-quality fresh fruits and vegetables are available year-round.

THE MACROBIOTIC MEAL

The ideal in macrobiotics is to serve at major meals one dish from each of these basic categories: soup, grain, bean and sea vegetables, cooked seasonal vegetables, salad, pickle, dessert, beverage. These may turn up in various forms: grains are considered the centerpiece of the meal, while the seasonal and sea vegetables could turn up in the soup, the salad, a side dish or an entrée. So could the beans. Both the pickle and the dessert are considered essential, in their own way, to digestion. The beverage is always drunk after, never with the meal. Typically it is *kukicha,* or roasted bancha twig tea.

For practical purposes I think it is a bit much to expect anybody to cook seven-course dinners immediately upon embarking on macrobiotics, unless that person has a great deal of time. As a way of getting into it, I have categorized the recipes as soups, grain dishes, bean dishes, vegetable entrées, side dishes, salads and desserts. Of course there is some overlapping. You might want to try to eat from at least two of these categories as a dinner at first—three, if you include dessert. Thus a dinner might be soup and a salad, soup and a rice dish, an entrée and a salad, soup and a side dish—plus dessert.

If you really want to experience proper digestion as the macrobiotic diet conceives of it, you will always start with soup and have a bit of pickle right after eating your entrées or salad and before dessert. You can do this without a good deal of trouble by keeping sauerkraut from the health food store on hand and eating about a teaspoon after your main course. Or eat part of a pickled umeboshi plum. If you want to eat soup, cook up a batch over the weekend that will last for several days, or keep one of the basic vegetable stocks (described in the recipe section for Stage Three) on hand in

---

DID YOU KNOW? Eating a simple broth before a meal is a standard weight-watching ploy. Macrobiotics teaches that it also stimulates digestion, and it is a great way to use up odds and ends of vegetables.

---

quantities in the refrigerator, and just add miso or leftover grain or beans and tamari and create "instant" soup.

Most macrobiotic desserts are so simple that they can be prepared during or even after dinner, to be followed with a beverage. Beverages are usually hot teas that have been allowed to cool somewhat, served unadorned.

As for water, controversy simmers among vegetarians as to whether spring water or distilled is better. The advantage of both is obviously their implied purity. The disadvantage of spring water is that, as with organic vegetables, you have no way of checking on the controls in its origins and handling unless you happen to be at the source. The disadvantage of distilled water is the same, plus the fact that if, as promised, it is chemically pure, it may have the effect of leaching desirable minerals out of your body without replacing them. Macrobiotic people tend to recommend spring water, calling distilled water "dead."

ONE DAY AT A TIME

If you aren't living up to the seven-course ideal in every dinner you cook, you may want to try to balance out your diet in terms of what you eat throughout the day. One habit that is helpful, though it may seem odd at first, is the macrobiotic practice of regularly eating miso soup for breakfast. This is often made with a stock containing wakame. In this way, you have already eaten miso and seaweed (wakame) before you know it. If you are still hungry, it can be followed with plain cooked oatmeal, with or without stewed fruit in winter or just fresh fruit in summer. Even by itself the soup is a great energizer, and is a filling dish to start the day. You can crumble a plain rice cake (Chico San makes them; get the unsalted kind) in it for extra body.

If you decide to try the soup route for breakfast, Basic Miso Soup from Stage Two is an easy recipe. Then as you go through the day, you can balance your diet with other foods at lunch and dinner. Grain and vegetables should be eaten every day, and more than once if practicable; sea vegetables and bean dishes should be eaten several times a week. Lunch should be coordinated with dinner if at all possible so that there isn't too much duplication.

For the time being, the grain at lunch could be bread, unsalted whole grain crackers (Ry-Krisp, Ryvita or Scandinavian flatbread) or rice cakes, eaten in the form of sandwiches or with spreads and/or salads. This is not too much of a departure from the standard American lunch, and is workable if you bring your lunch with you or have access to a health food or other reasonably good restaurant. You can make soup your lunch too—buy it or bring it from home and eat it with unsalted crackers, pita bread and/or salad. Another good lunch is leftover rice and vegetables, eaten cold or at room temperature. While non-yeast bread is preferred, pita pockets (look for the whole wheat ones) can be used for sandwiches or with soup some of the time. Toast them to make them more digestible and tasty—they'll swell up, too, making for easy stuffing. In salads, cooked or pressed salads are preferred to raw. Raw vegetables, because they are more Yin, are best reserved for the heat of summer. But if your health is good, you can bend the rules somewhat to suit your convenience and make the diet more approachable.

I mention health because many people turn to macrobiotics in the process of seeking to heal various ailments. If this is the case, one is pretty much expected to cooperate by observing the diet more strictly. The best thing to be doing in this instance is to work with a teacher who can make specific recommendations about specific health problems.

A macrobiotics teacher typically has studied at one of the East-West centers in the country, or perhaps under Michio and Aveline Kushi, the foremost authorities on macrobiotics in the United States. Many people consult a macrobiotics teacher for health-related reasons. Teaching includes explanation of the theory of macrobiotics as developed by George Ohsawa and others, and practical cooking lessons. A study of specific health problems may be included.

If a general improvement in health is what is sought, a fairly standard recommendation for proportions of foods to be eaten daily is: whole grains, 50–60 percent; seasonal vegetables, 25 percent; beans and sea vegetables, 5–10 percent; soups, 5 percent. Dessert, which might be served only at dinner, and beverage, which comes after the meal, sort of fit into the crevices.

One of the main tenets in planning a macrobiotic menu, besides including grains and beans and the less familiar seaweeds and soy foods, is the use of fruits and vegetables in season and according to climate. Thus for most of the United States, many popular and familiar foods become more or less out of bounds, including tropical and subtropical fruits—oranges, lemons, grapefruit, bananas, papayas, figs, pineapple and avocados—and the nightshade family—potatoes, tomatoes, green and red peppers and eggplant—which are considered too acid-forming and so not digestible. This may seem like hopelessly bad news, but there are plenty of new foods to explore, and the occasional use of citrus juice, eggplant or peppers is expected, if not encouraged. Dairy foods, meat and eggs are, of course, not part of macrobiotics, and for the most part they aren't missed. (Some macrobiotics folk use eggs occasionally.) Familiar spices are supplanted by new seasonings. The use of yeasted and soda breads is discouraged, but unyeasted and sourdough breads may be eaten in small quantities. Of course extreme foods are excluded—coffee, black tea, chocolate, tobacco, drugs and most alcohol, though beer or sake may be consumed occasionally and a cooking wine is used. The use of herbal teas is discouraged as too stimulating, but several other hot beverages are recommended. Refined foods and foods containing artificial preservatives, coloring or flavor are excluded. So are refined sugars and honey.

THE HYGIENIST MEAL

Hygienists separate starches, proteins and fruits, not eating any two of these at the same meal, and avoiding fats as much as possible.

The hygienists recommend making breakfast the fruit meal, lunch the starch meal and dinner the protein meal. While strict adherents believe that people would be best off if they ate only one food at a time and if they ate most foods raw, they recognize that we live in society and are prejudiced by our cultural upbringing to regard a meal as being something more than a quarter of a head of lettuce sitting on a plate. Charts and books available from the American Natural Hygiene Society in Tampa, Florida (see Resources) offer help in menu planning.

Before going any further it is well to note a few more hygienist caveats. Besides the rules of fruit only with fruit, no protein with starch or vice versa and no fat with protein or starch, avocado is considered to combine well with all foods except protein and melons; tomatoes can be eaten with non-starchy vegetables and protein, but not with starch (there goes spaghetti); and melons are always eaten alone. Condiments, especially salt and spices, are excluded. Dressings, including oil, vinegar and lemon, are frowned upon. Water and other beverages are taken alone, never with meals.

Desserts are generally forbidden. But, says Shelton, ever

DID YOU KNOW? Hygienists eat starches, proteins and fruits at separate meals, and avoid fats as much as possible. But they recognize that we live in society and are brought up to regard a meal as more than a quarter of a head of lettuce sitting on a plate.

the realist, "If you must have pie, have it alone and miss the next meal."

All that being said, standard hygienist fare may include fruit for breakfast; starch and green vegetables with green salad for lunch; and protein with green vegetables and salad for dinner. Among starches are included whole grains and starchy vegetables like potatoes, sweet potatoes and yams, winter squash and pumpkin, white dried beans and Jerusalem artichoke. Among things that count as green vegetables are the whole cole family, including cauliflower; summer squashes; okra; carrots, green peas and green beans; and the more obvious leafy greens. Proteins include nuts, dairy foods, eggs, bean sprouts, fresh corn, dried beans and flesh foods, which are eaten sparingly, no more than once a week. Avocados function as protein and as a green vegetable.

The greatest difficulty people initially experience in this diet is in separating their beloved starches and proteins, but it is basic to the diet. Another difficulty is doing without salt and cutting down greatly on fats. However, being gradually vegetarian will have helped on this one. Next, seeing all the salad on the menu, most people will recoil from the idea of eating it without any dressing (no acid with either starch or protein, and no fat with protein meals). If this seems hopelessly forbidding at first, I would suggest easing the transition by using very modest amounts of dressing made of the best-quality cold-pressed oil with fresh citrus juice or brown rice vinegar. I would also suggest eating the salad last in this case, so that the oil and acid enter the digestive system near the end of the meal, when digestion of the protein or starch has already had a chance to get under way. Fats, if eaten, may be offset by green vegetables, those great chlorophyll-bearing purifiers of the blood. That being so, you could sometimes make a lunch or dinner simply of salad with a buttermilk or cheese dressing—but then eat no starch or protein, besides what's in the dressing, for that meal.

I would also suggest starting lunch or dinner with a hot

soup, as macrobiotic dieters do. This could be a legume soup at meals where legumes are permitted. But for simplicity's sake, a simple vegetable stock can be made in quantity, and a little of it heated each evening, to serve as an "introductory course" at dinner. Or it may be taken along in a Thermos to work. Just bear in mind the hygienist dictum that liquid should be consumed fifteen minutes before the rest of the meal. I realize this may be difficult at work where lunch hours can be short and sometimes crowded, but if your soup is a stock, you can sip it from a cup at your desk fifteen minutes or half an hour before leaving for lunch or breaking out your brown bag. If your soup is a hearty one, such as a legume soup or barley-mushroom, treat it as one of your main courses and eat it with the meal.

Using a simple broth before a meal is a standard weight-watching ploy, since it takes the edge off your appetite, and it may be useful in adjusting to a diet bereft of some familiar comforts. And, as macrobiotic practice teaches, it stimulates the flow of digestive juices. It is also a great way to use up the odds and ends of the many kinds of vegetables in this diet. Just remember to include only odds and ends of "green" vegetables—no potatoes or other starchy vegetables.

Remember also that while the hygienists would probably prefer the simplest, least processed starch foods, whole grain breads, noodles and other pasta (including that made from Jerusalem artichokes) could be used as the starch in any given meal. The more processed a grain product, the more likely it is to be mucus-producing, and the wealth of plain whole grains—including rice, oats, barley and millet—shouldn't be forgotten, nor their partly processed counterparts—couscous, kasha and bulgur wheat.

In salads, tomatoes could be included in the protein meals, but not the starch ones. One hygienist source frowns on "irritating or bitter foods," including onions, garlic, parsley, endive, watercress and radishes. Shelton, however, allows cooked onions, and steamed garlic is equally mild, so these might be allowed in soups.

Of course, the hygienists' ultimate goal is fewer foods at a meal, not more. My recommendations are intended to make a transition period easier, should you decide to go this route. So is my final suggestion: use salt, unless you are on a salt-restricted diet. I know that the hygienists say it cannot be digested, but if you have been accustomed to the taste of it, going "cold turkey" may be enough to discourage you from sticking with a new diet. I suggest that you use as little as possible, and always make it part of the cooking process, since, as the macrobiotics practitioners suggest, this may make it more digestible. If you must use it on raw vegetables, roast it first. In a meal that includes nuts, you could use gomasio, the sesame-seed-salt preparation.

About shopping for and preparing hygienist meals there is not a lot to be said. Virtually all the ingredients are familiar, and the cooking is very plain. A few recipes from other regimens—notably the soups offered elsewhere in this book—can be adapted with a little thought, by eliminating any dairy foods and checking to make sure the other ingredients do not conflict. Minestrone, for example, would have to be adapted so that any given batch would include either tomatoes or beans or macaroni, but not in combination (no tomatoes with starch, not more than one starch at a meal; the dried beans do count as a protein sometimes, but also as a starch). For vegetables, starches and proteins, simplicity in cooking is the order of the day: boiling, steaming, baking, broiling and roasting.

About macrobiotics, however, there is a lot to be said, since many of the ingredients are unfamiliar. Let us consider what they are, where to get them, and what to do with them.

STAGE THREE:
NATURAL HYGIENE

The protein sources for a natural hygiene diet are much the same as those for Stage Two, with more emphasis on vegetable proteins (nuts, legumes) and less on animal proteins (dairy foods are eaten sparingly, and flesh food is recommended no more than once a week). The largely vegetable diet is high in vitamins A and C and in calcium and potassium. It is on the low side for B vitamins, and you should be careful to get enough of these.

The diet is also good for people in search of relatively bland meals high in fiber.

A day of hygienist menus could go like this:

Breakfast: sub-acid fruit (1 pear and 1 apple, diced) and yogurt (8 ounces).

Lunch: salad (lettuce, cabbage, carrots and green peppers), two green vegetables (1 cup cooked broccoli, 1 cup cooked summer squash), starch (1 cup cooked kidney beans, 1 cup carrot juice).

Dinner: salad (1 cup dandelion greens), two green vegetables (½ cup cooked kale, ½ baked eggplant), protein (1 cup cottage cheese).

GOOD NEWS:

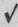 The yogurt, beans and cottage cheese combine to yield 57 grams protein, the adult male RDA. With the eggplant, broccoli, kale, and other vegetables, they also yield about 900 milligrams of calcium.

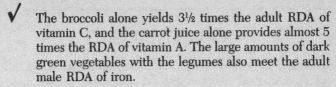

✓ The broccoli alone yields 3½ times the adult RDA of vitamin C, and the carrot juice alone provides almost 5 times the RDA of vitamin A. The large amounts of dark green vegetables with the legumes also meet the adult male RDA of iron.

✓ If you are trying to achieve a high-carbohydrate diet, eat more often, snacking on high-carbohydrate fruits and vegetables throughout the day. Just don't combine them. Again, the fruit juices are especially high in carbohydrates.

TAKE NOTE:

✓ A largely vegetable diet tends to be low in B vitamins. Look to fish of all kinds for these important nutrients. A pound of lobster might be your best buy for B_1, mackerel for B_2 and B_6, and crab for B_{12}.

✓ You may be surprised to learn that this fruit-and-vegetable diet is surprisingly low in carbohydrates (less than 200 grams for this day's meals). That's because it puts the emphasis on green and not starchy vegetables, and limits fruit to one meal a day.

FOOD COMBINING

In natural hygienism, meals are organized according to the principle of food combining. Food combining follows these rules for eating different kinds of food:

- ■ fruit with fruit
- ■ no protein with starch
- ■ no fat with protein
- ■ no fat with starch
- ■ green vegetables with protein or starch
- ■ melon alone

Possible meals following these principles are based on suggestions from the American Natural Hygiene Society. They follow this general pattern for a seven-day cycle:

Breakfast (summer): (1) melon; (2) berries with cream; (3) melon; (4) sub-acid fruit with yogurt; (5) sweet and sub-acid fruit; (6) sub-acid fruit with yogurt; (7) sweet and sub-acid fruit.

Breakfast (winter): (1) citrus fruit; (2) sub-acid fruit with yogurt; (3) sub-acid and sweet fruit; (4) sub-acid fruit with yogurt; (5) citrus fruit; (6) sub-acid and sweet fruit; (7) citrus fruit.

Lunch: salad plus two cooked "green" vegetables a day; one starch daily. Starches could include: (1) potato; (2) beans; (3) yams; (4) brown rice; (5) corn bread or wheat bread; (6) lentils; (7) millet.

Dinner: salad plus two cooked "green" vegetables a day; one protein daily. Proteins could include: (1) nuts; (2) cottage cheese; (3) avocado; (4) egg; (5) bean sprouts; (6) tofu; (7) fish.

FOOD CLASSIFICATIONS IN NATURAL HYGIENISM

Note that some foods can function in more than one category. They are listed in parentheses in their secondary category.

Proteins: nuts, dairy foods, bean sprouts, soybeans, avocados, all flesh foods, (cereals, dry beans and peas).

Starches: cereals, dry beans and peas, potatoes, yams, sweet potatoes, winter squashes, pumpkin, Jerusalem artichoke, and mildly starchy vegetables including cauliflower, beets, carrots.

Green vegetables: arugula, asparagus, beet tops, broccoli, brussels sprouts, cabbage, celery, chard, chicory, collards, cucumber, dandelion greens, eggplant, endive, escarole, garlic, green beans, kale, lettuce, mustard greens, onions, parsley, peppers, radish, spinach, summer squash, turnip tops, watercress, (beets, carrots, cauliflower).

Fats: vegetable and nut oils, butter and cream, (nuts, avocados).

Acid fruits: berries, citrus fruits, pineapple, tomato, pomegranate, (tart apples, grapes, peaches and plums).

Sub-acid fruits: apricots, cherries, figs, mangoes, papayas, pears, sweet apples, grapes, peaches and plums.

Sweet fruits: banana, sweet grapes, all dried fruit.

SOUP IDEAS

To add a hot soup for a starter to the hygienist meal, keep a simple vegetable broth made of green vegetables on hand and use it as a base for:

- a simple miso soup (no noodles) at protein meals
- a potato soup (compare Potage à la Bonne Femme, listed in the Index) at starch meals
- a bean, pea or lentil soup at legume meals
- a modified Ukrainian Borscht (no tomatoes) at starch meals (see Index for recipe)

FOURTEEN

SHOPPING AND COOKING MACROBIOTIC

Many of the staples of macrobiotic cooking are familiar and readily found at the grocery or health food store— brown rice, carrots, onion, broccoli, oats, dried beans, fresh fruits in season.

That's the good news. The bad news is that if your health food store doesn't carry certain essential ingredients, you are going to have to do some persuasive talking or find an additional source of supply. If you have been shopping at one store regularly, you may be able to persuade its owner or manager to try stocking a few of the things you need on a trial basis. The seaweeds keep almost indefinitely, and miso has a long shelf life, while tempeh can be stored frozen. Tofu is becoming increasingly popular in conventional cooking. These might be incentives to make a store more willing to keep on hand what you need.

For those who live in large cities, this will probably not be a problem, because there will be a variety of health food stores and very likely Oriental food stores. Fresh produce markets, Middle Eastern and even Italian groceries may be of help, too. The products in the Oriental groceries will probably not be labeled in English, but don't be afraid to ask someone to translate what's on the package.

If you live in an outlying area where the products you need are not available, you can locate the stores nearest you and make periodic trips to stock up. Let us consider how to stock the kitchen as efficiently as possible with familiar and new ingredients.

For the time being, think in terms of the variety available, how well it may be stored, and how it can be cooked. When the ingredients are more familiar and you have decided which ones work best for you, you can proceed to a more detailed study of their place in the macrobiotic diet.

GRAINS

Because they are considered the most balanced food in terms of Yin and Yang, grains have a special place in macrobiotic cooking. Ideally you should be eating grain at every meal, which means using all the grains we have already discussed, some of which are more familiar than others. In the most thoughtful macrobiotic meal planning, grains are varied seasonally. To some extent this is logical—corn is a summer grain, others like oats or rye are winter crops. And it is also somewhat in keeping with our own culture's habits—we are more likely to think of corn on the cob in summer and hot oatmeal in winter.

Certain grain foods are also considered nutritionally superior in the macrobiotic system—brown rice is said to be the most perfectly balanced food in terms of Yin and Yang, and as such is a kind of base by which all other foods may be measured. And whole grains are considered superior to those that are partly processed—whole grains are more complete than the cracked or partly processed grains like bulgur, kasha and couscous, which in turn are better than the more processed flour and noodles. And of course pastas and flour made from whole grains are better than more "refined" products. For the time being, use the grains interchangeably as they fit into your menu, not worrying too much about what to use when. Just strive for the best quality available.

By now you have certainly used brown rice in a number of meals—as a main component with stir-fry, fried rice, or with beans, perhaps in pudding; as a side dish with fish or moussaka. You can continue to use it in this way, and also—with the help of one of the seaweeds—create rice balls, an ideal lunch for brown bagging or traveling, and the more elegant sushi. Leftover rice can also be part of breakfast, tossed into a miso soup or heated and sprinkled with a little gomasio.

If you have been using the long-grain brown rice available in grocery stores, you should certainly try the medium- and short-grain rice sold in health food stores. Their fat kernels make a somewhat moister and stickier rice than long grain, which may also be obtained in health food stores. Experiment with the varieties. In macrobiotics, long-grain rice is more of a summer product, while short-grain is used in winter or for healing diets. Ideally, rice for macrobiotic meals—like all whole grain—is pressure cooked to enhance its nutritive value, which is an important consideration if you are going to be relying on grains for your protein.

Other grains that are most familiar to us are probably oats, rye, barley and buckwheat. Continue to use oats in their most familiar form—oatmeal—as a breakfast food. Try eating it unadorned, with just the salt it was cooked with for seasoning, and taste the goodness of the grain. Use it as an ingredient in breads and in soups for a thickener—either fresh dry oatmeal or leftover cooked oatmeal can be used in other cooked dishes. If you have a pressure cooker, try cooking the steel-cut oats instead of the more processed rolled oats or oatmeal.

Rye is used mostly in flour form, in whole grain breads. Barley is usually an ingredient in soups and stews. Buckwheat, besides its familiar form in kasha, is found in the

Japanese *soba* noodles. These fine slender noodles are excellent as a dish in themselves, or in soups.

Cracked or partly processed wheat like bulgur or couscous can be used interchangeably with kasha and with millet, which is a whole grain but has a similar texture to the cracked grains. For those who have eaten Southern cooking, the texture of all these grains will be reminiscent of hominy, the cracked corn product, but with much more flavor. Commercially available hominy is nutritionally an inferior grain, but if you like corn dishes, don't neglect stone-ground or water-ground corn meal in your health food store. Made into corn meal mush, as we Americans know it, or polenta, as the Italians call it, it makes good breakfast food.

Millet, valued in macrobiotics as the only alkaline grain, is considered especially good for people with an "acid" body condition. Make it into Millet-Vegetable Casserole (see Index), eat it plain for breakfast, or experiment by using it and the various cracked grains interchangeably (millet is fine in Tabbouleh, for example, which appears in the Stage Two Recipes).

Use any of the grains instead of rice sometimes, too. And use cooked leftovers in baking. Any of the cooked grains can be used instead of corn meal in a basic corn bread recipe, although the taste will be different with each grain. Or they can simply be added to yeasted or sourdough breads.

Whole wheat flour is the staple for breads. It is also an ingredient of the Japanese *udon* noodle, a fat, square noodle that is delightful as a main dish or in soups. Sourdough bread is available in health food stores and sometimes in specialty shops, or you can make your own. It hardens quickly unless kept frozen or refrigerated, and has a deliciously distinctive flavor and a chewy texture. Sourdough bread is preferred over yeast bread because it is considered more digestible—the yeast has a disruptively expanding effect in the digestive tract.

Rice, millet, wheat, barley, rye, oats and corn are the basic seven grains in macrobiotic cooking. Buckwheat is classed as a seed grass and not a cereal grain, but for practical purposes it is a grain, and an especially important one for people in cold climates because of its short growing season.

Grains have a long shelf life if kept in airtight containers away from heat and light. You should aim for the best-quality grains possible at this point, probably buying grain foods— even pasta—at the health food store. Soba or udon noodles will be available there, or in Japanese groceries.

Once the grains are cooked, they have a storage life in the refrigerator of a few days. It is better not to freeze cooked grains—it diminishes their nutritional value and ruins their texture. It's okay to freeze bread, especially sourdough bread —it is in fact the only way to keep it in quantity. If this seems contradictory, bear in mind that in the macrobiotic scheme of things, bread is nutritionally at the bottom of the heap.

In planning meals, the trick is to balance between having to cook whole grains every night, which is too time-consuming, and having too much left over to use it before it spoils. You might figure on cooking whole grain rice twice a week at first, and cooking enough each time for several meals. You can fill in at other meals with quicker-cooking grains, noodles and other pasta, bread and leftovers.

In general, you may find it works better for you to cook day by day, or to devote one day a week to making grain or bean dishes, soups, and other slower-cooking dishes in batches to be eaten throughout the week. The best practice is not to cook too far in advance, since fresher is better, but in a house where everyone works this may simply not be possible. Don't worry about it. Do what works and keep experimenting to improve the quality of your life.

BEANS AND OTHER LEGUMES

Legume dishes are recommended several times a week. That's not much, really, when you consider that beans include soy products like tofu and tempeh. You may find that you are eating beans and other legumes more often, since they make such a convenient centerpiece—meat substitute, if you will. Macrobiotic practitioners might eat whole beans several times a week, and other bean dishes—including tofu and tempeh—as desired on other days. Miso and tamari are not counted as dishes per se, incidentally. As ingredients in soups and many other dishes they are used every day.

Of the legumes, aduki beans are considered the best quality, but you will have to go to the health food store for them. Lentils and chick-peas are also considered good-quality legumes in terms of digestibility and nutritive value. Black soybeans are next; they also can be hard to find. Kidney, pinto, navy and soy beans, split peas, black-eyed peas and the black "turtle" beans used in black bean soup are eaten less frequently.

The earthy little aduki beans are especially digestible because of their low fat content. These and other beans will cause virtually no discomfort from intestinal gas if you cook them right. Soak aduki beans for four hours, others overnight. Discard the soaking water, rinse the beans, and cook them with a piece of the flat, chunky seaweed called *kombu* (more about that shortly) for several hours or until they are completely tender. The combination of the overnight soaking, discarding the soaking water and using the kombu renders the beans much more digestible. Use kombu with the quicker-cooking split peas and lentils as well, for flavor and digestibility.

Cooking beans and chick-peas is not a last-minute affair. There are shortcuts, including pressure cooking, but longer soaking does improve flavor and digestibility. So in any given week you may want to decide in advance whether the longer-cooking legumes will be part of the menu. You should try to include the aduki beans at least twice a month if not once a week. If the slower-cooking beans are on the menu, you'll have to schedule them for soaking overnight, followed by a day or evening where cooking them for a couple of hours won't make dinner hopelessly late. Or cook them in advance on a day off, or after dinner one night for use the next evening.

One week you might include only quicker bean dishes. A pound of tofu will last for several meals. Then a pot of lentil soup—a couple more meals—would round out bean dishes for the week. Or tempeh might make a meal or two, and a pot of split pea soup would round out the week. Another week, you might cook a pot of aduki beans—or aduki and kidney beans, or aduki and navy beans—at the beginning of the week and make several meals out of them. (When I cook them together, I usually give the larger beans a head start of about an hour, since the aduki beans seem to cook faster. This of course means soaking them separately.) Wait until the beans are tender, but not mushy, to add salt. Otherwise, as one teacher points out, they won't *get* tender. Then they should cook another twenty minutes. A pot of beans, cooked with kombu, onions and carrots, can go through the week—serve the beans with rice the first night; use them next in three bean salad; a third meal could include a bean soup using vegetable stock. Or leftovers could be mashed and seasoned to make a bean spread or even patties—bean burgers instead of lentil burgers.

SEEDS AND NUTS

By using gomasio, you will have sesame seeds on many dishes. And they're rich in protein and calcium, so that's good news for people who are concerned about getting enough of either. Other seeds and nuts can be used judiciously in stir-fry, stews, bean or grain dishes, salads, desserts—just about anywhere a little added texture and flavor are in order. Use them sparingly, however, because they are a rich, concentrated and often fatty food.

Sesame seeds are also the source of the preferred cooking oil, although corn oil may be used in baking. And sesame paste (tahini) is used with chick-peas to make Hummus, a great party dish or a meal in its own right.

SEASONAL VEGETABLES

The emphasis on things that are locally grown, and that grow naturally in your climate, does exclude the nightshades, for those of us in temperate zones. Even zucchini is frowned on in the strictest diets, but in common practice it is included for color and taste in mixed-vegetable dishes. Squashes and other "above-ground" and "ground" vegetables—including cucumbers and the whole cole or cabbage family—are considered excellent for the temperate climates, as are root vegetables and leafy greens, including watercress.

Try for a variety of tastes, textures and colors in planning your vegetable dishes, but again, if you are cooking for only one or two persons, don't overload the refrigerator with things that will wilt in a few days. This is actually less of a problem in macrobiotics than it might be in cuisines that use more delicate vegetables, since in macrobiotics most of the vegetables are pretty sturdy.

Two somewhat exotic vegetables that are mainstays of macrobiotic cooking are dried *shiitake* mushrooms and the *daikon* radish. Both are considered to play a role in discharging excess animal foods, fat and mucus from the body. Also, both are handy additions to your cooking repertoire because they last well and are flavorful. Finding them may be another matter, but if the health food store doesn't have them, the

DID YOU KNOW? A mainstay of macrobiotic cooking is the dried shiitake mushroom. Recently, fresh shiitake mushrooms have become a gourmet item in non-macrobiotic cooking as well. Look for them at fruit stands or markets that sell exotic produce.

Oriental grocery almost surely will. The shiitake is a dark brown mushroom that comes dried in packages. The daikon is a long white radish about the size of a very fat carrot. Both are frequently used in soups and stocks. The daikon, which can be cut and cooked in the same ways as a carrot, is good in just about any vegetable dish and often goes into pressed salads or pickle dishes. The shiitake must be soaked for a little while to make it tender before cutting. Recently, fresh shiitake mushrooms have become a gourmet item in non-macrobiotic cooking. Look for them at fruit stands or markets that sell exotic produce.

SEAWEEDS

This brings us to the biggest adventure in macrobiotic cooking—seaweeds, or sea vegetables, as they are often called. There are about half a dozen of these commonly used in beginning macrobiotic cooking, and some or all are frequently available in health food and Oriental stores. In the health food store you will find them packaged under familiar brand names like Eden or Erewhon. Ask for them by name in Japanese groceries.

Collectively, the seaweeds are high in iodine, calcium and other minerals, and contain vitamins A, B and C.

Nori comes in square, thinly pressed sheets that are used

in making rice balls and sushi. It can also be crumbled into soups. It is highest of the seaweeds in protein and in vitamins B and C.

Dulse is a reddish-purple seaweed that is highest in iron, and also fairly high in potassium and sodium. *Wakame* is a fan-shaped member of the kelp family that is very high in calcium. It and dulse are good in soups.

Kombu, another calcium-rich kelp, has been called "natural MSG" because of its flavor-enhancing qualities. It is used to make vegetable stocks and is also cooked with beans. Besides bringing out their full flavor, the kombu makes them more tender, more digestible and less gas-producing. It is an indispensable item if you are planning to depend on legumes for much of your protein.

Kanten, also called agar-agar, is a translucent, chunky seaweed sold in strips or flakes. Dissolved in liquid over heat and then allowed to cool, it jells, providing the basis of desserts or aspics. It is recommended for dieters because it contains no protein, fat or carbohydrates. It contains some calcium and a trace of iodine.

Other seaweeds commonly used in macrobiotic cooking are *hiziki* and *arame.* Both are used in salads and vegetable dishes. Hiziki's fine dark strands have a pleasing texture and mild flavor. Arame can be cut up to resemble hiziki.

Any other seaweeds—including Irish moss and members of the kelp family—that you find in the health food store can be used in soups or vegetable dishes. In recent years, Americans have begun cultivating and harvesting seaweeds, especially from the rocky New England coast. But some varieties are still imported from Japan.

Minerals and enzymes in seaweed are considered valuable in helping the body adjust to a vegetable diet. It has also been reported that the brown algae, including wakame, kombu, hiziki or arame, help the body discharge heavy metals—including radioactive wastes—from the intestines, in the form of insoluble salts. The active ingredient in these seaweeds is alginic acid. It may be that experiments with seaweed, reported in *East-West Journal* and elsewhere, have accounted for the upsurge of interest in sea vegetables among Americans in recent years.

In any case, they are a useful source of calcium for people who are eating less dairy food. They cook quickly and easily; just soak them for a few minutes first, then cut them up, if necessary, and add to whatever dish you are cooking. Kanten and kombu don't need soaking; just add to the liquid you are heating. And nori can either be crumbled, dry, into soups, or toasted over an open flame or burner.

OTHER EXOTICA

There are various condiments and seasonings you can start using if you don't already do so. Tamari, miso, gomasio and fresh ginger, which is often available in supermarkets nowadays, are probably already familiar.

Brown rice vinegar, which is mild and delicious, is preferred to any other vinegar; Eden is one brand name available in health food stores. Don't give up till you've located some and tried it—after which you will be thoroughly spoiled and want to use nothing else. It's good for salads and as a flavoring for the stronger leafy greens, like cooked collards or kale. Mirin, a Japanese cooking wine, is available in health food stores.

Umeboshi plums are another unfamiliar item for most people. They can be used, a pinch or two at a time, for your after-dinner "digestive aid" pickle. Also called salt plums, they *are* actually a kind of pickle. They are soft and easily mashed into a paste that is used in dressings. They are also an ingredient for rice balls and for a tea that is used as a sort of tonic if you are feeling fatigued.

Among sweeteners, barley malt syrup and Yinnie syrup—made of rice and other grains—are preferred to honey or sugars. They are less sweet and are used sparingly in desserts. Both are available in health food stores. Maple syrup may be used occasionally, but be sure it is pure maple syrup. Barley malt and maple syrup will both mold, and should be refrigerated. Along with the sweeteners goes the thickener *kudzu*, or kuzu, made from the root of the kudzu plant, which is cluttering up woods and highway cuts throughout the South. So pesky is this plant that it even gave its name to an obnoxious comic strip character, so it's nice to know it has its uses. Kudzu is cooked to dissolve in liquid, and then begins to congeal, making it ideal for preparing puddings, glazes or thickened sauces. (Arrowroot is also acceptable, but kudzu is said to have digestion-aiding properties.)

Other unfamiliar products include the staple beverage, made from roasted tea twigs and called *kukicha*. It is also referred to as roasted bancha tea or just bancha tea. There is a green bancha tea, but it should be avoided because it contains caffeine. Barley "coffee" (one brand is Wilsons Heritage) and barley tea (*mugicha*) are all right. Beverages are not drunk until the meal is over, since it is held that the liquids interfere with digestion by diluting the digestive tract's secretions.

FRUITS AND OTHER SWEET THINGS

The role of fruits is almost exclusively to serve as part or all of a cooked dessert. Seasonal fruits and berries—apples, peaches, blueberries—are used to complement dinner, and their sweetness is considered to slow down the digestion process, signaling to the digestive system that the meal has ended.

It is the nature of sweet things to be very Yin, and too much Yin is not considered good for the overall health of the individual. So sweets are eaten sparingly, and they are usually cooked, to render them more Yang (the application of heat causes foods to contract, though they may first go through a stage of expansion). Fruits can be cooked quite deliciously by stewing or baking; they can become sauces or compotes; they can be cooked and then "jelled" using kanten, or made into a pudding with kudzu root. Occasionally either of these may be used to fill a crust made with flour and oil. Cookies or a macrobiotic Brown Betty or fruit crunch are also good occasional desserts.

COOKING

There are many fine points to macrobiotic cooking, and I will deal with some of these in individual recipes. In general, remember that if you are going to use salt in a dish (of course it should be sea salt), it should be added during cooking— usually toward the end, so it won't toughen whatever you are cooking, but before the active cooking process is finished. Also remember that salt flavoring may be imparted from miso, tamari, gomasio and the seaweeds. Taste before you season. Onions are always started ahead of whatever other vegetables they are cooked with, to drive off their volatile oils. When cooked, onions become sweet and also more digestible.

Remember to use oil sparingly in cooking.

In proper macrobiotic preparation, even the arrangement of vegetables in a cooking pot is done according to the principles of Yin and Yang (excepting the onions, which always go first), so that the more Yin elements will rise from the bottom of the pot and the more Yang elements will descend from the top. This is rather technical at first, however, and for starters you may simply want to add ingredients as common sense and the recipe dictate.

UTENSILS

This is the last, but not at all the least, consideration in setting up a macrobiotic kitchen. With good basic tools you may already have on hand, you are well on the way: heavy pots, a good cutting knife and board, wooden spoons. You need a kettle for soups and a wok or large frying pan for sautéing. Basically the utensils recommended in Stage One will stand you in good stead.

However, there are some specialized tools you may want to acquire, gradually or all at once. If you are going to adopt macrobiotics for good, you'll need a stainless steel pressure cooker for grains. This can be obtained at many department stores or through catalogues. So can a Foley food mill for puréeing soups and sauces. Oriental stores and some health food stores can provide bamboo twig mats for rolling sushi; a plastic salad press; suribachi mortar and pestle for grinding gomasio; a heavy carbon steel cleaver for vegetables; a ceramic ginger grater and a bamboo tea strainer (conventional counterparts will do as well). You'll also want a whetstone for the knife, which you can find in the hardware store.

Flea markets and secondhand stores can also be good sources of tools. I got my chopping board and a set of good iron skillets at a flea market, for $4 and $3 respectively. My Foley food mill was $3 at an "antiques" shop. But I would buy the pressure cooker new; you want to be sure it is working properly, and be able to exchange it if need be. Besides, most of the secondhand ones are aluminum, and you don't want your vegetables to be absorbing aluminum leached into the cooking water.

STAGE THREE: MACROBIOTICS

The protein, vitamin and mineral sources in a macrobiotic diet include foods not familiar to Western tables. A macrobiotic vegetarian still counts heavily on grain and legumes for essential protein, but among the legume foods are the soybean products—tamari, tofu, miso and tempeh. These are also rich in various vitamins and minerals, as are the seaweeds: nori, kombu, dulse, kelp, hiziki, arame and wakame. Fresh-cooked vegetables and fruits are also emphasized.

Because of its emphasis on grain and legumes, the macrobiotic diet is high in carbohydrates as well as protein.

A day of macrobiotic menus (see Index for specific recipes) could include:

Breakfast: 1 cup Miso Soup, 1 cup oatmeal with raisins and cooked apples.

Lunch: Rice Balls, leftover Pumpkin Soup.

Dinner: Onion Soup, Beans with Rice, Vegetable Sauté, Hiziki with Carrots, Kanten with Fruit (peaches).

This day's menu provides about 74 grams of protein, thanks to the rice, beans, miso, oatmeal, seaweed, bonito flakes (in the Pumpkin Soup) and vegetables and fruits. Its carbohydrate yield is a high 330 grams. Vitamin A content is 1½ times the daily requirement, and vitamin C slightly more than the RDA; these are supplied by the cabbage, carrots and watercress in the Vegetable Sauté, and by the other vegetables, fruits and seaweeds. B vitamins and iron are supplied adequately by the seaweeds, miso, bonito, grain, and beans.

GOOD NEWS:

✓ One serving of tempeh (4 ounces) supplies an estimated 60 percent of the RDA of hard-to-find vitamin B_{12}, plus 30 percent of the RDA of vitamin B_2 and 8 percent of the RDA of B_1.

✓ Besides the amounts of B vitamins supplied directly in macrobiotic meals, the body's supply of these vitamins is further enriched by the action of fermented foods in the digestive tract, where more B vitamins are manufactured. The macrobiotic diet is rich in fermented foods: tamari, miso, tempeh, natto and all the pickled dishes including umeboshi plums.

✓ The seaweeds are a rich source of minerals. For example, 3½ ounces of hiziki provides 1,400 milligrams of calcium (almost twice the RDA) and 29 milligrams of iron (10 milligrams more than the adult female RDA).

✓ For dieters, kanten (available in health food stores) provides a sweet treat that is low in calories. The kanten itself, which is virtually calorie-less, is mixed with apple juice, other unsugared fruit juice, or cooked fruit, and jelled in the refrigerator. A 4-ounce serving provides as much as 400 milligrams calcium and 5 milligrams iron as well!

FIFTEEN

PUTTING IT ALL TOGETHER

When I try to envision a family tree of vegetarianism, I see widely divergent branches. Yet their common roots are evident—a desire to take more control of one's eating habits and not just leave them to chance or Madison Avenue; a growing interest in traditional ethnic foods; a growing abundance of tools, ingredients and information.

In the interests of exploring all the possibilities that may make it easier for someone to be a vegetarian, we have looked at some possibilities that a fruitarian or strict vegetarian might reject, including hygienism and macrobiotics. But in their strictest forms, these are both purely vegetarian diets. In their more popular form, they, like lacto-ovo-vegetarianism, are a transition for former meat eaters.

THE RECIPES

If you look back over recipes we have already worked with, you will see that many of them may be adapted quite simply to macrobiotic cuisine, by omitting dairy foods and sometimes adding new ingredients here and there. For soups, experiment with new vegetable and seaweed stocks, and omit dairy products and the nightshade vegetables. Add seaweed and daikon for nutrition and zest. For casseroles, substitute tofu for cheese in the dish, and use a little white Miso Sauce instead of Parmesan on top. Stir-fry goes right ahead—without meat, of course, but with chunks of tofu if you like.

Tempeh, as we know, is a substitute for those who still miss the texture of ground meat. Using it, you can take vegetarian chili one step further by omitting tomato—a nightshade vegetable, remember—and the characteristic chili spices, which of course are too spicy for macrobiotic cooking. Instead you can flavor your bean-and-tempeh dish with onions, celery, daikon radish, grated ginger and soy sauce.

In learning to omit dairy foods, you will find that quiche can be made without eggs—use tofu instead—and while the binding effect of eggs in patties (like lentil burgers) and baked goods is convenient, it is not necessary. As for the nightshades, use grains where possible instead of potatoes, substitute other vegetables for peppers, use eggplant occasionally, and learn to omit tomatoes, whose flavor you should find clashes subtly with macrobiotic meals anyway.

There are also new recipes and suggestions for Stage Three, by way of further introducing macrobiotic cooking. People frequently turn to macrobiotics as a healing diet, and if that is your purpose, the recipes in our Stage Three section may serve to help you integrate macrobiotics into your cooking and eating habits.

Macrobiotic meals, as we noted earlier, proceed in an orderly fashion from soup to pickle, with perhaps a bit of dessert and a beverage to cap the meal. Our dishes in the recipe section are presented in that order—soups first, then main dishes, side dishes and salads, dressings and condiments, desserts and beverages.

Even if you decide not to pursue macrobiotics, you can certainly profit from knowing how to use the protein-rich tempeh and tofu; the kudzu can usefully be transferred to any recipe you know; the kombu can be cooked with all legumes to make them more digestible; the shiitake mushrooms can be used to make a delightful broth base for soups. By now, of course, some of the early recipes in the book may not be applicable to your eating style. But if you go back, you'll see that with minor changes, many of them can be adapted and updated. The Mulligatawny Soup from Stage One, for instance, can be converted to a non-meat base simply by using any of the macrobiotic stocks instead of chicken broth.

A table of the recipes in the Appendix is for quick review and help in your menu planning.

MENU PLANNING

As you may recall from Stage One, I am not enamored of the idea of people following weekly menu plans laid out to the last cracker by someone else. Part of the point of shopping for staples is to have enough components on hand so that you can be flexible. But the other side of shopping is to stock up on the perishables that are going to fill in this week's meals. Put them together and it does add up to menu planning.

The main thing to keep in mind is not to overdo one area and neglect another. Some suggestions:

■ Use the recipe table to remind you of possible dishes you may have forgotten.

■ Try to get input from family members when you make up the weekly shopping list—what do they want to see more or less of?

■ Take one week in which you write down what the family eats for breakfast, lunch and dinner. Analyze it for variety and nutritional value. Don't overuse favorite or "easy" meals.

■ Adapt the recipes from Stages One, Two and Three to suit your needs and tastes, and apply ideas from these recipes

—especially the ideas of freshness and digestibility—to your own favorite recipes.

THE INDIVIDUAL COUNTS

In the last few chapters, we have seen how the paths of various vegetarians can diverge. But in the end, they all twine back together again, and the direction they are taking, as we can see if we stand still and look for a moment, is toward self-sufficiency.

In learning to think consciously about our eating habits, we see how we may discard those that do not serve us well. We may also become aware of the larger implications of the food we eat: where it comes from, whether it represents an efficient use of raw materials, and whether in fact we really either need or want it. We have a powerful opportunity to vote with our food dollars, for as they go, so flows the food market.

All around the country, people are finding innovative ways to healthier eating. From New York City comes the story of a family of five who dine on macrobiotic meals for well under $100 a week in food bills. What's more, they don't cook it themselves. Because the parents work, they pay a vegetarian cook $10 an hour to prepare a week's worth of meals to be stored in the refrigerator and heated up by "whoever gets home first"—including the three teenage children.

In Orlando, Florida, a determined mother of three small children caught the *Orlando Sentinel*'s attention when she decided that it was *not* too much trouble to make baby food from scratch. "Until the age of six months," the *Sentinel* reported, "the babies were nursed and then were gradually introduced to solid puréed foods, freshly harvested from the Parrishes' backyard garden and processed through a baby-food grinder. To Mrs. Parrish, a food grinder is essential to making your own baby food. There are several kinds available, all small enough to fit in a handbag and resilient enough to last through three babies." The food was steamed or otherwise cooked before processing and then thinned with milk or other liquid. The children spurned commercially prepared baby foods and went on to become toddlers who preferred snacks of cucumber or broccoli to candy and junk food.

The point is, the individual can and does make a difference. We need to think about what we can do, individually and collectively, to make our lifestyles more self-sufficient from the standpoint of our food supply. And our food supply, let's not forget, is intimately connected to our national energy supply, to the depletion of natural resources including the soil, and to the world food supply.

Whether we are looking for someone to cook us macrobiotic meals or for the nearest food co-op, what we need is a network. Good places to look locally for information are the community bulletin boards at grocery stores, churches, schools and colleges. Community colleges or local adult schools may even offer courses on the subjects you're looking for.

In addition, there are national publications and groups that can provide useful information. These and a list of basic source books are offered in the Resources section.

The possibilities might be modestly individual, such as growing your own vegetables or supporting your local farmers by buying their produce whenever possible. Or they might be individually ambitious, such as constructing your own root cellar or studying aquaculture. Or they might take the form of group effort like starting a food co-op, or the grander global strategy envisioned by Frances Moore Lappe's Food First Institute, an effort to end world hunger by education and collective action. It is not beyond our means to help take the pressure off the world's dwindling resources, and perhaps discover a new and better lifestyle for ourselves in the process.

THE
GRADUAL
VEGETARIAN

RECIPES

SIXTEEN

RECIPES FOR STAGE ONE

FOR STARTERS, SOUP

Soup is traditionally a first course, although the Romans liked to start with eggs. In many societies, soup is also a meal in itself. Macrobiotics nutritionists recommend soup as an opener because a simple dish like vegetable-based hot broth accelerates proper digestion, while cold foods tend to inhibit the digestive process.

In the interest of promoting simpler meals, hearty soups can be a meal in themselves or go with salad or a sandwich for an everyday supper. The word "supper" in itself is revealing of the French custom of taking the larger meal at midday (customarily followed by a rest) and a simple meal in the evening—*le souper*. It was while living with Annie Nicole and her family in eastern France that I learned the habit of dining on a thick soup of puréed vegetables, usually with a carrot-and-potato base, which took little time or fuss to prepare and was eaten with a simple salad of garden greens and plenty of fresh bread and sweet butter. That soup is commonly rendered in this country as Potage à la Bonne Femme.

We are so brainwashed about meat that we tend to assume that all soups start with a meat broth base, preferably made from scratch. This simply is not so; from the standpoint of flavor, many vegetable soups stand nobly on their own. And luckily so, since preparing a meat broth takes at least a couple of hours, while many vegetable soups can be made from start to finish in an hour or less—including the following Potage à la Bonne Femme, Spinach Vichyssoise (a relative of Potage à la Bonne Femme), and two kinds of minestrone.

POTAGE À LA BONNE FEMME

An excellent winter supper with black or rye bread.

4 medium potatoes	Pinch of basil, thyme
1 carrot, finely sliced	and/or rosemary,
1 cup shredded cabbage	crumbled
1 medium onion,	1 tablespoon butter
chopped	4 peppercorns
Celery rib and leaves	salt to taste
	Yogurt (optional)

Put 4 cups of water on to boil. Wash and slice the potatoes and the carrot, both with skins still on. Shred or slice the cabbage; chop the onion, celery and—if fresh—the herbs.

To the boiling water, add carrot, potatoes, onion, butter, peppercorns and a teaspoon or more of salt (the potatoes soak up a great deal).

Cook half an hour, or until potatoes can easily be pierced with a fork. Add cabbage, celery and herbs and cook 20 minutes. Put the cooked vegetables through a food mill or blender, or beat the soup for a couple of minutes with an egg beater. The texture should be almost but not quite a purée.

Correct seasoning and, if you like, add 1 tablespoon of plain yogurt for each serving of soup. *Makes 2–4 servings.*

SPINACH VICHYSSOISE

An excellent hot soup for cold winter evenings. Chilled, it's great for summer suppers.

2 tablespoons butter	1 tablespoon salt
6 medium potatoes, scrubbed	10 ounces fresh spinach, washed and drained
1 medium onion, chopped	3 tablespoons yogurt
1 carrot, chopped fine	Black pepper

Melt butter in a heavy kettle and add potatoes, onion and carrot. Sauté for a minute, then add 2 quarts water. Bring to a boil, add salt, and cook until vegetables are tender, about half an hour. Add spinach and cook a minute or two, until wilted. Purée in a blender, food processor or food mill, or use an egg beater. The consistency should be mealy, not quite smooth. Return to the kettle. Thin with water or milk if too thick. Stir in yogurt. Garnish with freshly ground black pepper. *Makes 6–8 servings.*

MEATLESS MINESTRONE

It's really the beans, the greens, the tomatoes and the pasta that give minestrone its taste and texture, and not the meat. You'll never miss it. Good for crisp fall evenings with real Italian bread or pumpernickel and red table wine.

1 cup dried split peas	¼ teaspoon basil
1 large onion, chopped	1 bay leaf
3 small potatoes	2 pinches of thyme
1 pound can of tomatoes	2 or 3 peppercorns
	1 clove
½ teaspoon oregano	2 carrots, chopped

¼ head of cabbage,
  sliced
½ pound spinach or
  escarole, chopped
1 cup cooked or canned
  kidney beans or
  chick-peas

1 cup cooked macaroni
Salt
Yogurt or grated
  cheese

Rinse the split peas. Put in a kettle with 2 quarts water and bring to a boil. Boil for 30 minutes and add onion, potatoes, undrained tomatoes and the herbs and spices (not the salt). Cook until potatoes are soft and peas begin to disintegrate. Add carrots and cook until tender. Add cabbage and spinach. Cook for a few minutes, add beans and macaroni, and cook for 10–15 minutes, adding more liquid if needed. Season with salt to taste. Garnish with a teaspoon of yogurt in each bowl or with grated cheese, if desired. *Makes 6–8 servings.*

NOTES: Improves the second or third day; more liquid may be needed on reheating.

Other vegetables may be added: chopped celery, cooked corn, sliced squash, chopped green peppers.

GENOESE MINESTRONE

This minestrone is a re-creation of the steaming bowls of soup we used to get at the Bleecker Street Luncheonette (now called Pietro's Home Cooking) in New York's Father Demo Square. The thing that made this minestrone exceptional—and it did seem to be the best in the world—was that it contained virtually no tomatoes. Its base was split peas.

½ cup split peas, washed
  and drained
2 tablespoons olive oil
1 medium onion,
  chopped
1 garlic clove, minced

½ small zucchini squash,
  sliced
1 cup chopped escarole
  or spinach, washed
  and drained

½ cup cooked or canned white or kidney beans
1 celery rib, chopped
1 tomato, quartered (optional)
1 bay leaf
1 teaspoon oregano
1 cup cooked macaroni
Salt and pepper
Parmesan cheese

Bring split peas and 1 quart water to a boil. Heat oil and sauté onion and garlic. Add other vegetables and herbs—the tomato last—and sauté briefly. When the peas are falling apart, about 30 minutes after they start to boil, add the sautéed vegetables and cook another 15 minutes. Add the cooked macaroni, taste, and season with salt and pepper. Serve with Parmesan cheese. *About 4 servings.*

LENTIL MUSHROOM SOUP

1 cup dried lentils
2 peppercorns
2 carrots, scrubbed and thickly sliced
½ pound mushrooms, cleaned and sliced
1 medium onion, sliced thin
1 tablespoon oil or butter
Tamari sauce or salt

In a deep kettle, bring 1 quart water to a boil and add lentils, peppercorns and carrots. Cook half an hour, or until nearly tender. Sauté mushrooms and onion in the oil and add to the lentils. Cook until the lentils are tender, but not mushy, adding more water if needed. Season with tamari or salt to taste.

Serve with dark bread. *Makes 6–8 servings.*

SPLIT PEA SOUP

Serve with a good dark or rye bread or with grilled cheese sandwiches for a hearty supper. Made in large batches, it will last for several meals.

1 tablespoon butter	2 cups split peas, rinsed and drained
2 medium onions, chopped	Salt or tamari sauce to taste
3 peppercorns	Grated cheese, chopped peanuts or yogurt
2 carrots, sliced	
1 celery rib, chopped	
1 medium potato, washed and sliced thin	

Melt butter in a large kettle; add onion, peppercorns, carrots, celery and potato. Cook until onions are translucent and add 1 quart water. Bring to a boil and add peas and 1 teaspoon salt. Bring to a second boil, reduce heat, and simmer 30–40 minutes, until peas are soft and separating from their skins. Add water during cooking if the soup appears to be getting too thick or boiling away. When peas are soft, purée, using a blender, food mill or rotary egg beater. Adjust for seasoning and thickness, adding more water if necessary to obtain a soup that is smooth but not thin. Both the peas and potatoes absorb a lot of water and salt, and the amounts of water and salt needed will vary with the batch of soup and with personal taste. You may need 2 quarts water.

The soup should not be too finely puréed. A slightly mealy texture from the bits of vegetables is ideal. Garnish with grated cheese, chopped peanuts, or a teaspoon of yogurt per bowl. *Makes 6–8 servings.*

BARLEY MUSHROOM SOUP

A hearty soup, good with dark bread for a winter supper.

2 cups barley	½ pound or more
Salt	mushrooms, cleaned
1 medium onion,	and sliced
chopped	1 tablespoon oil
1 carrot, sliced	Tamari to taste
thin	Scallions (optional)

Rinse barley and bring to a boil in 2 quarts water. Add a dash of salt, reduce heat, and simmer 40 minutes. Meanwhile, sauté onion, carrot and mushrooms in oil. Add to barley after 40 minutes and simmer another 15 minutes, or until barley is tender. Season to taste with tamari and cook 5 minutes more. Garnish with chopped scallions, if desired. *Makes 6–8 servings.*

QUICK CHICKEN-CORN CHOWDER

This is a two-step dish. It is actually a way of using leftover bones from a stir-fry with chicken or other dish that requires boning. What I do with those bones is to set them to boil immediately in a few cups of water, until the remaining shreds of meat have come off the bones and the broth is golden. Then I store or freeze the broth with the bits of meat in it until I need it for the chicken chowder.

1 cup dried noodles	1 celery rib, chopped
3–4 cups chicken stock	½ onion, chopped
with meat	½ carrot, sliced
1 cup fresh or frozen	Salt and pepper to
corn kernels	taste

Handful of spinach
leaves, washed,
drained, and cut
into ribbons

Cook the egg noodles in 2 cups boiling water. Heat the stock; add the corn, celery, onion and carrot. Cook 10 minutes. Add the cooked noodles and season to taste. Add the spinach ribbons, cook a minute or so, and serve. Garnish with parsley or chopped hard-boiled egg. *Makes 4 servings.*

MULLIGATAWNY SOUP

Another good use for the leftover bones and scraps of chicken from stir-fry, a roast, or what have you. A delicious Indian soup.

1½ quarts chicken stock (see below)	2 small apples, sliced
1 medium onion, chopped	2 medium tomatoes, quartered
1 garlic clove, chopped	2 tablespoons oil
1 carrot, chopped	1 tablespoon Basic Curry Powder (recipe follows)
1 celery rib, chopped	
½ green pepper, chopped	1½ cups red lentils, rinsed
1 turnip, chopped	Chopped parsley

THE STOCK:
Boil bones and scraps of leftover raw or cooked chicken until the broth is pale gold and the meat falls off the bones. Use about 2 quarts water to start, with 1 teaspoon salt and a couple of peppercorns. When stock is ready, remove the bones. An easy way to do it is pour the broth through a colander. Pick out the bones and return meat to the broth.

THE SOUP:
Heat stock to a boil. Sauté the vegetables and apples in oil with curry powder until the tomatoes start to fall apart. Cook lentils and vegetables in broth half an hour or more, until tender. Pureé in a blender or with an egg beater. Garnish with parsley if desired.   *Makes 6–8 servings.*

BASIC CURRY POWDER

3 teaspoons turmeric	½ teaspoon cayenne
1 teaspoon cardamom	pepper
1 teaspoon coriander	½ teaspoon ginger
1 teaspoon cumin	

All the measurements are for ground dry spices. Blend and store in a cool dry place.

SALAD DAYS

Salads can be a side dish, the centerpiece of a meal, or one course in an extended repast, but for heaven's sake, let the salad assume its proper importance in the meal. Keep the side dish salads very simple—just one or two kinds of greens —so that they'll be convenient to fix; let the fancier salads be a main dish, not just an appetizer.

For side dish salads, try combining a soft-leaf lettuce with a stronger type of green, such as escarole, spinach or mustard greens.

Salade Niçoise and Caesar Salad are ideal for the really hot weather. Each is a meal in itself, and the preparation won't overheat the cook or the kitchen.

EASY GREEN SALAD

Why is this an easy salad? Because none of the ingredients is especially perishable, and so you're likely to have them on hand. Also because the dressing is as simple as possible. This is a good salad with a basic pasta dinner.

½ head romaine (or other) lettuce, washed, drained and torn up
Handful of cabbage shreds
Handful of chopped celery, ribs and leaves

Small handful of broken nut meats
1 carrot, shredded
Oil and vinegar (or lemon juice)
Salt and pepper

While dinner's cooking, clean and cut up the vegetables and nuts and toss together in a bowl. Just before serving, dribble oil over the salad, using just enough to coat the leaves. (Don't drench it.) Toss until leaves are coated. Sprinkle lightly with vinegar or more liberally with lemon juice, add salt and pepper, toss and taste. Correct seasoning. *Serves 3–4.*

NOTES: Add any other raw greens you like to the lettuce mixture. Escarole and spinach are good additions.

An easy way to drain the lettuce is to tear the leaves first, then wrap in a clean dish towel and swing in tight circles to force the water out of the lettuce. (This is best done in the bathroom or out on the back porch unless you don't mind getting a spray of water all over the kitchen.)

It is best not to use metal implements on lettuce, because they bruise the delicate leaves and mar their flavor. Tear the leaves instead of cutting them, and use wooden spoons or salad implements to toss the salad.

CAESAR SALAD

In summer it's a meal in itself, with French bread on the side.

1 head romaine lettuce	Parmesan cheese
1 garlic clove, halved	Salt and pepper
2 egg yolks	Toasted sesame seeds
½ cup olive oil	(optional)
Juice of 2 lemons	
Garlic Croutons	
(recipe follows)	

Wash and drain the lettuce. Rub serving bowl with garlic; discard garlic. Separate egg yolks from whites (discard whites or save for use in baking). Tear lettuce and toss with oil. Add yolks and toss to coat lettuce leaves. Add lemon juice and croutons and toss. Add cheese, salt, pepper and sesame seeds if desired, and toss. *Serves 4.*

NOTE: Traditional Caesar salad recipes call for anchovies. I find the sesame seeds make a good substitute for those who dislike anchovies or don't want to be bothered with a tube of paste or a can of anchovies when all they need is one anchovy fillet.

GARLIC CROUTONS

Instant croutons in case you don't have the traditional stale bread handy.

1 slice of bread per person	1 garlic clove
	1 tablespoon oil

Toast the bread and cut into crouton-sized pieces. Sauté the garlic briefly in oil, add croutons, and stir until they are lightly coated with oil. Remove garlic and use croutons for salads or soups.

TACO SALAD

A do-it-yourself Tex-Mex-style salad bar. Good with rice and beans or lentil soup.

  6 taco shells

THE FILLING:
   Shredded lettuce, cabbage and carrots
   Sliced onion
   Sliced tomatoes
   Chopped scallions
   Sliced green pepper
   Sliced avocado
   Grated cheese

THE DRESSING:
   Oil
   Vinegar

Salt
Pepper
Tabasco sauce

Set out all the ingredients and let people stuff and dress their own tacos. *Serves 3–4.*

Low-fat Egg Salad

An old favorite for lunches, minus the mayonnaise.

4 hard-boiled eggs
½ cup small curd cottage
     cheese
¼ cup chopped celery
1 tablespoon lemon
     juice
Salt
Pepper

Mash ingredients together in a mixing bowl. Spread on whole wheat bread and top with salad greens and/or alfalfa sprouts. Or serve plain, atop romaine lettuce leaves. *Makes 4 sandwiches.*

Salade Niçoise

An ideal summer supper, this is a complete meal in one dish that requires minimal use of the stove and may be made in advance. It is festive enough for guests and may be augmented with a good French, Italian or sourdough bread with sweet butter and a dry white wine for special occasions.

1 cup cooked and
     cooled string beans
4 hard-boiled eggs,
     sliced
4 small potatoes,
     cooked, cooled and
     sliced
Lettuce leaves

Basic Vinaigrette
Dressing (recipe
follows)
2 medium tomatoes or
handful of cherry
tomatoes, sliced

1 can tuna, drained
1 medium onion, sliced
Olives

Cook the beans, eggs and potatoes in advance—the night before, if you can—to let them cool. Get a couple of handfuls of fresh beans if available, snap them and boil 5–7 minutes. You can boil the beans, eggs and potatoes all in the same pot if you want to save effort and energy—the eggs should be left in about 10 minutes, the potatoes until they pierce easily with a sharp fork. Used canned beans if fresh aren't available.

To assemble the salad, line a large bowl with lettuce leaves. Add the potatoes and string beans and douse with one third of the dressing. Add tomatoes in a layer, followed by the tuna, the sliced egg, the onion and the olives. Add the rest of the dressing. *Serves 4–6.*

BASIC VINAIGRETTE DRESSING

½ garlic clove, mashed
⅓ cup olive oil
⅓ cup vinegar (wine or
cider)
Dash of honey

¼ teaspoon dry mustard
Salt and pepper to
taste
Basil or parsley, if
desired

Combine ingredients. Taste for balance of oil to vinegar and correct proportion if necessary. May be made in larger quantities and saved.

SALAD DRESSINGS

These all derive from the basic vinaigrette given with the recipe for Salade Niçoise. You can adapt the basic recipe or its cream version, Yogurt Dressing, with herbs and spices of your own choosing, and with avocado, blue cheese, curry, or what have you. If you use a lot of salad dressing, make it in quantity and store in the refrigerator. If the oil congeals, let it liquefy at room temperature before serving.

Alternate vinegar and lemon juice at will. Use only good-quality oil: sesame for a light dressing, olive oil for a Mediterranean effect, a nut oil occasionally if you like. Here are some favorite variations.

YOGURT DRESSING:

To the Basic Vinaigrette (see Index), add 1 or 2 tablespoons plain yogurt and mix well, to provide a light but creamy dressing.

YOGURT-SESAME DRESSING:

To Basic Vinaigrette (see Index), add 2 tablespoons yogurt, ½ teaspoon herb or herbs of your choice—dill, basil, thyme or marjoram are good—and 1 tablespoon lightly toasted sesame seeds. The sesame seeds give the dressing a rich flavor.

FRENCH DRESSING:

To the Basic Vinaigrette (see Index), add ½ teaspoon dry mustard and 1 teaspoon paprika. Shake or mix well before serving.

MUSTARD DRESSING:

To Yogurt Dressing (see Index), add 1 tablespoon dry mustard and 1 teaspoon extra honey. This one is especially good on a salad containing bitter greens.

CUCUMBER DRESSING:

To the Basic Vinaigrette (see Index), add 2 tablespoons yogurt and 1 cucumber, peeled and seeded. Add a fresh mint leaf or two if available. Purée in a blender or force through a sieve. Excellent on hot days, when salad might be a meal in itself, or with Middle Eastern meals.

CONFETTI TUNA SALAD

1 6½-ounce can tuna,
    drained
2 tablespoons plain
    yogurt
½ small onion, chopped
½ celery rib, chopped
½ carrot, chopped
¼ teaspoon dried thyme
    Juice of ½ lemon
    Black pepper
1 teaspoon mayonnaise

Mix ingredients, adding extra yogurt or lemon juice if needed
for a moister salad. *Makes about 3 sandwiches or 2 healthy
servings on lettuce.*

TUNA MELT

With the soup of your choice, this makes a quick and filling
supper.

3 English muffins
    Confetti Tuna Salad
    (see Index)
¼ pound Cheddar
    cheese, sliced thin

Spread the muffins with tuna salad and top with enough
Cheddar cheese to cover the tuna mixture. Put under broiler
for several minutes, until bubbly. *Serves 2–3.*

INFINITE VARIATIONS ON POULTRY

Poultry offers so many possible entrées that whole cookbooks have been written about them. You doubtless already have favorites, and may find some old friends here in new guises, as well as new acquaintances. And don't overlook the obvious roast—chicken, turkey, guinea fowl, duck, or even goose. The chicken especially does not have to be for a festive occasion, and does not require a time-consuming stuffing. Instead, put a peeled onion or lemon slices in the body cavity, and roast as basic directions indicate, usually 20 minutes a pound in a medium oven.

Most of the following recipes specify chicken because it's the most familiar and is available in a variety of combinations of cuts. Other poultry may be used as well; each has its own flavor and texture.

MEG HERRON'S PARMESAN CHICKEN

1 fryer, cut up	½ cup Parmesan cheese
3–4 tablespoons melted butter	½ cup flour

Dip chicken pieces in melted butter and then in Parmesan cheese (the packaged variety, like Kraft, not fresh cheese, is what we're talking about here) mixed with flour.

Bake at 400 degrees for about an hour, or until tender. If cheese starts to burn, cover with foil for remainder of baking time. *Serves 4 or more.*

NOTE: Oil may be used instead of butter or mixed with the butter.

BAKED SESAME CHICKEN

A handsome and tasty dish for company, courtesy of Susan Greatorex. Nice with rice and fresh string beans.

2 chicken breasts, split	1 tablespoon sesame
1/3 cup tamari	seeds
1/3 cup sherry	
1 teaspoon ground ginger	

Place chicken, rib side down, in a baking dish. Mix tamari, sherry and ginger and pour over chicken. Sprinkle with sesame seeds. Bake 45 minutes at 350 degrees. Baste once or twice, being careful not to dislodge seeds.   *Serves 4.*

CHICKEN MARSALA

Serve on a bed of brown rice, surrounded by plain steamed vegetables to offset the richness of the Marsala sauce. Broccoli and carrots, steamed, make a pleasing color contrast.

1 frying chicken, cut up (or 2 breasts and 4 legs)	1/4 cup oil
	1/4 cup soy sauce
	1 cup Marsala or sherry (more as needed)
2 garlic cloves	
1/2 teaspoon dried ginger, or 1/2 inch fresh ginger, minced	1 teaspoon butter
	1 pound mushrooms, cleaned and sliced

Cut breasts into quarters and separate legs into thighs and drumsticks.

Sauté chicken, garlic and ginger in 3 tablespoons of the oil, turning chicken on both sides. Add soy sauce and continue to sauté until the soy sauce begins to coat the chicken like a glaze. Add Marsala, cover and simmer over low heat until tender, about 20 minutes.

While the chicken is simmering, heat remainder of oil and the butter in a second pan and quickly sauté the mushrooms, until they begin to give up their juices. Add to the chicken for the last 5 minutes of cooking. If the chicken needs more liquid during cooking, add more Marsala. *Serves 4–6.*

CHICKEN SHISH KEBAB

A good dish for a picnic. Or serve it at table on a bed of rice.

2 chicken breasts, boned	2 peppers
½ cup tamari	1 dozen cherry tomatoes
½ cup lemon juice	2 medium onions
¼ cup oil	8 mushrooms, minus
1 garlic clove, mashed	stems
1-inch piece of fresh	
ginger, grated	

Cut the chicken into bite-size pieces and marinate with tamari, lemon juice, oil, garlic and ginger for at least an hour or as much as a day, refrigerated.

Just before cooking, clean the vegetables and cut the peppers and onions into bite-size pieces. Thread chicken and vegetables onto four skewers, alternating to form a pleasing contrast of colors and flavors. Cook over a charcoal fire or under the broiler, basting with the marinade. *Makes 4 or more servings.*

NOTE: Use this recipe for any firm-fleshed fish, or for scallops.

STEWED CHICKEN PAPRIKA

A one-dish meal that can be ready in about an hour. Good for workday evenings, and a real mainstay in winter. This is our adaptation of Selwyn Ryba's mother's chicken, with many thanks for countless evenings of dining pleasure.

3 onions, quartered	Oil
2 celery ribs, chopped	2 garlic cloves, chopped
1 tomato, chopped	
1 green pepper, chopped	Paprika
	Salt and pepper
8–10 carrots, chopped	¼ teaspoon basil
4 medium potatoes, sliced thin	¼ teaspoon thyme
	1 bay leaf
1 whole chicken, cut up	

Bring 2 quarts of water to boil in a large kettle. While it is heating, clean and chop the vegetables. Sauté chicken in oil and garlic, sprinkling with paprika, salt and pepper as it cooks lightly on both sides.

Add chicken to the kettle and cook for half an hour. Add the onions, celery, tomato, green pepper, carrots, potatoes, basil, thyme and bay leaf, and cook for 20–30 minutes.

Serve in large soup bowls or in plates with a good raised lip, with plenty of broth. If desired, serve bread on the side for dipping.   *Serves 4.*

NOTE: This is a good recipe for including other root vegetables if you want to vary it and try out their flavors: rutabagas are especially nice; turnips or parsnips can go in, too. You can also add thinly sliced cabbage during the last 5 minutes or so of cooking. The tomato can be omitted if you don't have one handy.

Chicken Paprikash

This makes a nice dish for family or company. It goes well with noodles, over which it is served in Hungary. A traditional side dish is raw cucumbers and onions marinated in a vinaigrette dressing for a few hours at room temperature. Serve with pumpernickel bread, sweet butter and white wine for festive occasions.

1 frying chicken, cut up	Paprika
1 cup flour	1 cup water or white
Salt and pepper	wine (more if
¼ cup cooking oil	needed)
1 garlic clove, minced	

Dredge the chicken in flour, salt and pepper. Heat the oil in a large heavy skillet and sauté the garlic. Add the chicken, sprinkling liberally on both sides with paprika as it cooks. Brown lightly on both sides, add liquid, cover and simmer over low heat for half an hour, or until chicken tests tender when pierced with a cooking fork. Check during cooking and add more liquid as needed. *Serves 4.*

Notes: There is no substitute for Hungarian rose paprika if you can get it. But it can be hard to come by, and if you can't get it without trouble and expense, the grocery store paprika makes a tasty dish. Paprika has a tendency to develop its own variety of mealy bugs if kept too long, so be sure to cover tightly when not using. Paprika is rich in vitamin C.

The noodles traditionally served with chicken in Hungary are homemade nockerln or dumplings, but if you don't have the time or inclination to make your own, use store-bought egg noodles.

DONNA RICHARDS'S POT PIE

In this pot pie—a pot pie in the traditional sense—the dough is not on top in a crust, as we're accustomed to find it in commercial pot pies. It is a sort of cross between noodles and dumplings, cooked in broth. The broth is a good way to use up chicken or turkey bones from a roast after the meat is mostly gone.

THE BROTH:

1 chicken or turkey carcass	1 carrot, chopped
	1 celery rib, chopped
2 quarts water	3 peppercorns

THE DUMPLINGS:

2 large eggs	Flour, sifted
3 tablespoons butter	

Make the broth by boiling the chicken or turkey bones in the water until the broth is golden and the meat separates from the bones. Add the carrot, celery and peppercorns to the pot. After the meat is off the bones and the broth is cool enough to handle, pick out the bones and discard. Set the meat aside. Then you're ready to cook the dumplings.

Break eggs into a large mixing bowl. Add butter and mash it into small lumps, mixing it with eggs. Add enough flour to make a fairly stiff dough, one that you will be able to handle on a floured board. Turn it out onto a floured surface, dust it with flour, and roll out a little dough at a time, using a clean, lightly greased rolling pin that has been dusted with flour. Roll out the dough (a small handful at a time, remember) until it is almost translucent, and cut it into 2-inch squares. Clean knife blade frequently. Drop the dumplings, a few at a time, into simmering broth, until all are cooked—they will be a little puffy and pale gold and will float when done. Return meat to broth. Serve in shallow soup plates. *Makes 4–6 servings.*

NOTE: The only difficult thing about this recipe is the dough. If you haven't had much experience with dough, read the section on baking first. And in any case, you'll get it right with a little practice. Just remember to take small portions of dough each time, to use flour to prevent sticking to the board or rolling pin, to stop and clean off the rolling pin and knife— if necessary even wash and dry them—if the dough starts to stick. The worst thing you'll get is dumplings that are a little on the heavy side, and they'll get lighter every time you make them.

CHICKEN PARMIGIANA

1 whole chicken, cut up
  Flour, salt and
  pepper for
  dredging
	8 ounces sliced
	  mozzarella or other
	  light cheese

¼ cup oil	4 ounces Parmesan cheese, freshly
3–4 cups Basic Marinara Sauce (see Index)	grated

Dredge the chicken lightly in flour and sauté in oil until barely golden. Arrange in a baking dish, cover with marinara sauce, and top with cheeses. Bake in a 350-degree oven for 20–30 minutes. Serve with spaghetti and a tossed salad. *Serves 6.*

NOTES: Sliced leftover chicken or turkey may be used without the dredging and sautéing, for a dish that is not so rich.

Other variations:

Dip the chicken in a light batter (2 eggs beaten with 1 tablespoon flour and ¼ cup water)—this makes a heavier dish.

Vary the amount and variety of cheeses for a lighter or heavier dish.

Top-broil until cheese is melted instead of baking, if you are in a hurry. If you use this method, sauté the chicken until tender, adding ½ cup water to insure thorough cooking. Then add the marinara sauce and cheese and top-broil 5 minutes.

This recipe may be used with jumbo shrimp as well. Allow 3–4 per person.

EASY ROAST CHICKEN

This chicken without stuffing requires virtually no effort, and gives you the aesthetic effect of carving a bird without the time needed for a larger fowl. It will take longer than an hour to fix, of course, but gives you the dividend of possible leftovers—depending on how many mouths there are to feed—and the bones and scraps for soup. For a more elaborate bird, see Stuffed Chicken on following page. Serve with rice and a salad or side vegetable.

1 3–5-pound roasting chicken	1 onion, peeled
Salt	½ lemon, sliced
Oil	Thyme

Rinse and drain the cavities of the chicken and rub with salt. Rub outside with oil. Stuff large cavity with onion, lemon and a large pinch of thyme. Roast at 450 degrees for 10 minutes, then turn down to 350 and roast until done. Allow 20 minutes per pound. *Serves 4 with leftovers.*

NOTES: If pan gravy is desired, heat the roasting juices quickly on top of the stove, stir in 1–2 teaspoons flour, and dilute with water and a squeeze of lemon juice.

For moister, more tender meat, roast chicken breast side down for the first half of the cooking time.

ROAST STUFFED CHICKEN

Follow directions for Easy Roast Chicken, on preceding page, but fill both cavities with the following:

3 cups stale bread crumbs or croutons	1 small onion, minced
¼ cup milk	1 celery rib, chopped fine
1 egg	1 tablespoon sage
¼ cup melted butter	1 teaspoon thyme
¼ cup yogurt	¼ cup chopped walnuts

Toss all ingredients together thoroughly and stuff chicken. Allow up to 5 minutes more per pound to cook. If you are cooking the bird upside down for part of the time, secure the stuffing in the large cavity by covering it with aluminum foil for the first half of the cooking. In any case, secure the neck cavity with toothpicks or by sewing down the flap of skin. Stuffs a 5-pound chicken.

NOTE: If the bird comes with giblets, these can be boiled to make stock, and the liver chopped and added to the dressing.

CHICKEN WALDORF SALAD

I was never a great fan of Waldorf salad, but this variation is delicious. It's a fine party dish, good for buffets and picnics, or for light luncheons or suppers in summer. A real crowd pleaser.

1 pound seedless white grapes, halved	½ cup broken walnut meats
2 large apples, chopped	3 celery ribs, chopped

Juice of 1 lemon
1 whole roasted chicken
   or equivalent, diced
¾ cup mayonnaise, more
   or less

¾ cup yogurt, more or
   less
1 tablespoon Toasted
   Sesame Seeds
   (recipe follows)

Combine the fruit, nuts and celery, and toss with lemon juice to prevent the apples from discoloring. Add chicken, mayonnaise and yogurt and toss gently. (It is a good idea to start with half the indicated amount of both, and add more only as needed.) Garnish with toasted sesame seeds if desired. *Serves 6–8.*

NOTES: Friends report they have used this as a recipe for leftover turkey with great success.

Winesap apples are nice and tart if available.

TOASTED SESAME SEEDS

Rinse whole sesame seeds and drain. In a heavy hot skillet, toast them over medium-high heat, shaking the pan at intervals, as for popcorn, to prevent burning. After the water from the rinsing evaporates and they begin to toast, they will start to pop, like popcorn. When a fair number start to pop, the seeds are done. Don't toast too thick a layer or the seeds on the bottom will start to burn before the seeds in the middle are dry.

Store in refrigerator.

TANDOORI CHICKEN

From India, a chicken dish that is tangy and spicy and is especially delicious cooked over charcoal. Serve with rice and cucumber salad.

1 frying chicken, cut up

THE MARINADE:

- 1 cup plain yogurt
- 2 cloves crushed garlic
- ½ teaspoon cayenne pepper
- 1 teaspoon ground ginger
- 1 teaspoon cardamom
- 1 teaspoon coriander
- 1 teaspoon cumin
- Juice of 2 lemons

Mix the ingredients for the marinade, pour over chicken, and marinate for several hours. Bake or barbecue the chicken. *Serves 3–4.*

NOTE: For those who aren't eating fowl, try this recipe with any firm-fleshed fish.

FRUITS OF THE SEA

People who live within a hundred miles of the ocean really do have an advantage. Fresh fish is a delight—fillets can be pan-broiled or broiled or baked with a little butter and lemon, or steamed with herbs. But frozen fish is tasty, if not delectable, in the recipes that follow. Freshwater fish may be substituted by those fortunate enough to have access to them. Fresh clams, mussels and oysters are often available at some inland markets. Otherwise you will have to rely on frozen scallops and shrimps. While shellfish are very expensive, the recipes that include them are based on the certainty that a little goes a long way when they are combined with other ingredients, as in paella and bouillabaisse, creole and curries. Paella and bouillabaisse, incidentally, are not hard to make but are certainly more time-consuming than the average meal and also more expensive. They are included because they are glamorous crowd pleasers.

Most of these recipes are simple and basic. Fish is delicate and does not lend itself to prolonged cooking. And it seems a shame to obliterate its flavor with strong sauces.

STEAMED FISH

This is an especially good way to cook a dark oily fish because the steaming expresses the oils out of the fish, leaving it mild and much more digestible. Steaming can, of course, be used with any fish. Goes well with brown rice and steamed broccoli and carrots.

1 pound fillet of bluefish, weakfish, or other fish	2 garlic cloves, sliced thin
1 lemon, sliced thin	Crushed basil and chopped parsley

Use a fish steamer, or rig one by turning a vegetable steamer upside down in a large pot or skillet. A bamboo steamer will work too, if you have one. Grease whatever portion of the steamer the fish will come in contact with to avoid sticking. Lay the fish on or in the steamer, skin side down. Arrange the slices of lemon and garlic so that the top of the fish is completely covered, and sprinkle liberally with the herbs. Then place the fish over ½ cup or more of water in the pot or steamer and cover. If using a pot, steam on top of the stove until tender when pierced clear through with a fork. If using the fish steamer, cook in a 325-degree oven until done, about 7 minutes. Cooked fish, if done perfectly, is tender but does not disintegrate when cut and served; it may be flaky if it is a white fish, but is not dry. The dark fish will remain moister and hold together better. Dark fish takes longer to cook than light. *Serves 3.*

PAN-POACHED FISH

Serve on a bed of brown rice, with steamed vegetables or a salad.

1 tablespoon butter	Paprika
1 pound fillet of flounder or other mild fish	Chopped parsley
	Juice of 1 lemon

Melt the butter in a large heavy skillet, preferably not an iron one, since it will mar the delicate flavor of the fish. Add fish and sauté over medium heat without turning until the fish begins to turn white. Sprinkle with paprika and parsley and cook, covered, for several minutes, until fish is tender when poked with a fork. Add lemon juice just before serving. *Serves 2–3.*

WITH SCALLOPS:

Melt the butter. Add ½ pound bay or sea scallops. Cook, turning, until they start to brown slightly. Then push aside, add the fish, and proceed as above. *Serves 4.*

NOTES: This dish may be made in the oven when larger quantities are needed. With the scallops, it is an ideal dish for entertaining. Add a half cup of white wine at the outset for greater moistness.

Put the fish and the scallops together in a lightly greased dish. Dot with butter and sprinkle with paprika. Bake at 350 degrees 5–10 minutes, or until fish is flaky and scallops are tender. Garnish with parsley and serve on a bed of rice.

TUNA STEAKS

These rich, firm fish steaks have about as much to do with canned tuna—not to demean that handy substance—as fresh salmon does with its canned counterpart. Once you discover them, you'll wonder where they've been all your life.

4 fresh tuna steaks	3 tablespoons butter
Flour for dredging	Juice of 2 lemons
Salt	2 lemons, quartered
Pepper	

Dredge tuna in flour, salt and pepper. Melt butter in a heavy skillet and cook the tuna until lightly browned on both sides. Add lemon juice and cook a minute or two longer. Garnish with lemon wedges. *Serves 4.*

NOTES: Salmon and swordfish steaks work with this recipe, too.

Tuna and salmon steaks may also be grilled under the broiler or over charcoal. The latter is especially delicious. If you decide to grill or broil the steaks, omit the flour dredging, and baste with 2 parts lemon juice to 1 part oil—olive oil is good—or just with lemon juice.

GRILLED BLUEFISH

Ideal for picnics, served with fresh corn and a salad.

¼ cup olive oil Juice of 1 lemon 2–3 tablespoons Dijon mustard 1 large garlic clove, chopped	Fresh or dried basil, sage, thyme or other herb 1 pound fillet of bluefish or weakfish

Combine oil, lemon juice, mustard and garlic. Chop or crumble herbs into the marinade. Lay the fish on a large platter and pour marinade over it, lifting fish to be sure marinade coats the underside as well. Let stand several hours before cooking.

Turn once or twice. Cook the bluefish over charcoal or under the broiler for at least 10 minutes on each side, using the marinade as a basting sauce. For added flavor when grilling outside, spread a bed of fresh or dried herbs over the coals just before starting the fish. To prevent fish from sticking, cook in a well-greased hamburger-holder set on top of the grill. *Serves 2–3.*

SEA BASS WITH BLACK BEAN SAUCE

To prepare this elegant dish, which originated in the kitchen of Philadelphia food writer Elaine Tait, you must have access to an Oriental food store that sells fermented black beans.

While you're there, you might want to pick up the thin, translucent rice vermicelli to make a bed for serving the fish. Sake—for cooking and with the meal—is optional. Steamed snow peas (fresh ones are available at many grocery stores) are excellent on the side.

2 fillets of sea bass (about 2 pounds)	2 tablespoons sake or sherry
2 tablespoons oil	¼ teaspoon black pepper
2 tablespoons fermented black beans, mashed	1-inch piece fresh ginger, grated
2 tablespoons tamari	4 scallions, chopped

Rub the fish with oil on both sides. Lay fish on a steamer rack, or on a plate, and set in a pot with a tight-fitting lid. Spread black beans over fish.

Combine tamari and cooking wine and pour over fish. Sprinkle with pepper, ginger and scallions. Cover bottom of pot with water, making sure that there is not enough to touch the fish. Cook over medium-high heat or in a 350-degree oven until fish is very tender when pierced with a fork, 5–10 minutes. *Serves 4.*

SHRIMP CREOLE

A savory dish and fancy enough for company. Serve over rice, with cooked greens or a green salad on the side.

2 medium onions, chopped	Olive oil
3 garlic cloves, chopped	1 large can (16–20 ounces) tomatoes
1 bay leaf	1 tablespoon filé powder (see note)
1 large bell pepper, chopped	1 pound shrimp, cleaned and deveined
1 hot pepper, chopped, or ¼ teaspoon cayenne pepper	Red wine

Sauté the onions, garlic, bay leaf and sweet and hot peppers in oil until onions are translucent. Add the tomatoes, reserving juice. When tomatoes begin to disintegrate, add the juice and the filé powder, and simmer over low heat for about half an hour, adding red wine or a little water if necessary to keep the sauce liquid. Add shrimp and cook 5–7 minutes more, until shrimp are done. *Serves 4.*

NOTE: Filé powder is a traditional Creole seasoning made from sassafras root. If you can't find it or don't want to bother looking, a reasonable substitute can be made by combining 1 teaspoon coriander and 1 teaspoon cardamom. You may also find sassafras tea in a health food store; you can use it, with the cardamom and coriander, to approximate filé powder. If you are using loose sassafras root, bark or leaves, tie it up in a bit of cheesecloth so you can remove it after cooking.

PAELLA

This is not a quick dish, but excellent for entertaining. Everything up to the rice can be done in advance.

4 chicken breasts, quartered	1 tablespoon coriander
4 chicken legs, separated	1 tablespoon oregano
2 garlic cloves	4 cups brown rice
Olive oil	1 large pinch of saffron
Paprika	2 peppercorns
2 medium onions, chopped	1 pound shrimp
1 large green pepper, chopped	1 dozen clams or other shellfish
1 hot pepper, chopped (optional)	1 cup baby peas (fresh, frozen or canned)
	Chopped pimientos or sweet red pepper (optional)

Sauté the chicken pieces with garlic in oil, sprinkling with paprika. Meanwhile, bring 2 quarts water to a boil. Add chicken to water and let simmer.

Sauté onions, green pepper and hot pepper with coriander and oregano in the skillet that contained the chicken. Add this mixture, including the oil, to the simmering pot. Add the rice, saffron and peppercorns and simmer, covered.

(Note: If you are preparing this dish a day or even hours ahead, do not add rice at this point. You want to serve the dish with the rice freshly cooked so that it doesn't get gummy. So if you're preparing in advance, pause with the chicken getting tender. Resume about an hour before you plan to serve. At that point, rinse the rice, bring the pot to a boil, add the rice and start cleaning the shellfish.)

Clean shrimp and scrub clams. Keep an eye on the pot, adding more water if needed. When rice is nearly tender, put shrimp, clams and peas in a skillet with water to cover the bottom of the pan (or juice from the peas, if canned). Cook over medium heat 5–7 minutes, until shrimp and peas are done and clams are open. Arrange chicken and rice mixture on serving platter and pour shellfish and peas over it. Garnish with pimientos or sweet red peppers, if desired. *Serves 8 or more.*

NOTES: If you can't get fresh seafood, use frozen shrimp and any other seafood you like and can get—canned crab, lobster or clams, smoked oysters, frozen scallops. The shellfish is really just for effect and a bit of flavor. Don't feel you need a lot of it.

I suggest canned peas in this case as an exception to the canned-food moratorium because it is important that the peas be small and sweet.

PASTA

Pasta is a key step in the transition to vegetarianism because we think of it as an entrée, although the Italians don't. Among the main dishes that can give you meatless meals, with a minimum of preparation, are Linguine with White Clam Sauce, Pasta Primavera and Ratatouille. A basic Marinara Sauce is also indispensable, served plain over pasta or as a key ingredient in other pasta dishes.

PASTA PRIMAVERA

This is a delicate combination of flavors and textures—the sweetness of the carrots and nuts, the sharpness of the tomato and celery, the piquancy of the garlic, the crunchiness of the vegetables against the softness of the pasta. The vegetables must be fresh, except for the tomato, which may be canned. This dish has enjoyed great popularity at *nouvelle cuisine* restaurants. The secret to easy cooking at home is to prepare all the vegetables by cleaning and cutting in advance of the cooking. Serve over buttered pasta—a thin spaghettini or fettuccine goes well.

3 tablespoons butter or sesame oil
1 cup milk
1 green pepper, julienned
1 tablespoon fresh basil, or 1 teaspoon dried
Pinch of thyme
2 small carrots, sliced and cut into matchsticks

3 garlic cloves, chopped
½ small onion, chopped
1 cup chopped broccoli or other dark green vegetable
1 tomato, coarsely chopped
½ cup chopped celery, rib and leaves
1 medium summer squash, julienned

6 fresh mushrooms,
   sliced
¼ cup broken walnut
   meats
1 tablespoon flour
2 teaspoons grated
   Parmesan cheese

¼ cup yogurt
Freshly ground
   pepper and salt to
   taste

Heat the butter or oil and the milk in separate pans. Put the vegetables on to steam in a steamer in a large pot with a lid, starting with the slower-cooking pepper, herbs, carrots, garlic, onion and broccoli. Add the tomato, celery, squash, mushrooms and nuts after the other vegetables have cooked 3–5 minutes. To the butter, add flour, stirring, then the hot milk to form a very light white sauce. Turn off heat under the sauce and stir in the cheese and the yogurt. Serve the vegetables on top of pasta, add salt and pepper, and cover with the sauce. *Serves 2–3.*

EASY PASTA PRIMAVERA

A quicker version of the classic primavera, devised one weekend at a beach house equipped with only a skillet and a large pot, plus an assortment of odds and ends from the local farmers' market.

⅓ pound linguine or
   other pasta
2–3 tablespoons butter or
   light oil
½ small zucchini, finely
   chopped
6 large mushrooms,
   sliced
1 small onion, finely
   chopped

2 garlic cloves, finely
   chopped
½ medium pepper,
   finely chopped
1 egg
   Grated cheese
1 large tomato

Cook pasta in boiling water. When it is half done, heat the butter in a skillet and dump in all the vegetables except the tomato. Stir-fry on low heat, stirring steadily. When they begin to give up their juices, set aside.

By now the pasta should be done. Drain, rinse in cold water and return to low heat, stirring till steaming. Remove from heat, toss in the egg and cheese to coat the pasta lightly, and set aside.

Return vegetables to the stove, and quickly cut up the tomato and add, stirring over a medium to high flame until the tomato pieces lose their shape and blend in. Serve at once over pasta, with additional cheese if desired. *Serves 2.*

RATATOUILLE

This mainstay of Provençal cooking is exotic, easy to fix, and very cheap in summer. It expands to feed multitudes and is pretty enough to serve company. It goes well over pasta with a tossed green salad on the side, or with French bread and red wine for festive occasions.

1 medium eggplant, sliced thin
  Salt
2 garlic cloves, chopped or crushed
1 medium onion, chopped
1 green pepper, chopped
¼ cup oil (preferably olive)
1 medium zucchini, sliced
1 yellow squash, sliced
1 teaspoon dried basil, or handful of fresh chopped basil
1 teaspoon dried oregano, or ½ teaspoon thyme or rosemary
1 large can (28 ounces) tomatoes, juice drained and reserved
  Red wine

Lay the eggplant slices on paper towels to drain after salting them lightly. Sauté garlic, onion and pepper in the oil in a large skillet or Dutch oven. Add the eggplant and sauté until soft. Sauté the squash with the rest of the mixture until it starts to brown, add herbs and then tomatoes and wine, and simmer until the tomatoes have begun to break down, stirring as needed to prevent sticking. Serve over pasta of your choice, topped with grated cheese if desired. *Makes 6 or more servings.*

NOTES: It is common to salt eggplant before cooking and let it sit for 10–15 minutes to draw out some of the large volume of water it carries. The draining also takes away a slightly bitter taste. Since the eggplant takes a while to drain, it is a good idea to slice it first and set it to drain, then cut up the other vegetables. This way the eggplant is drained when you're ready to add it to the recipe. Salt watchers may drain their eggplant by steaming it, as is done in the next recipe.

Tomato paste may be added to this recipe for a thicker sauce. Or the ratatouille may be added to leftover marinara or spaghetti sauce.

EASY SUMMER RATATOUILLE

A good way to use up the bounty of your garden—or your neighbor's. Exact amounts aren't given because of the bounty problem (ask any squash grower). Just use roughly equal amounts of eggplant and squashes and as many tomatoes as you feel like or have on hand.

Figure on about 1 medium onion, 1 green pepper and a couple of cloves of garlic per quart of vegetables. That's liquid quarts.

Eggplant, sliced	Yellow squash, sliced
Zucchini, sliced	Onion, chopped

Garlic, chopped or
crushed
Green pepper,
coarsely chopped
Oil (½ olive, ½
sesame is good)
Fresh tomatoes,
coarsely chopped

Herbs to taste (fresh
basil and thyme if
available)
Salt and pepper to
taste

For lighter summer cooking, render the liquid out of the
eggplant by steaming it first instead of salting it. Meanwhile,
sauté the squashes, onion, garlic and pepper together in
enough oil to coat them lightly.

Add the eggplant, tomatoes, herbs and salt and pepper.
Cook until the tomatoes break down somewhat and the other
vegetables are tender. An elegant-looking dish because of its
bright colors. May be served over pasta with grated cheese or
eaten with pita bread. *Makes as much as you can stand!*

NOTES: Leftover ratatouille goes well over toast, topped with
a Basic Cheese Sauce (recipe follows), for a kind of Mediterranean Rarebit. Or use the leftovers in Ratatouille-Tofu
Lasagne (see Index).

In making the ratatouille or other sauces with fresh tomatoes, I don't usually bother to skin or seed them. You can skin
them by dipping them briefly in scalding water; the skins will
peel right off. But it isn't necessary at all.

BASIC CHEESE SAUCE

1 tablespoon butter
1 cup milk
1 tablespoon flour

½ cup (or more) grated
cheese

Melt butter in saucepan. Heat milk to boiling in a separate
pan. Add flour to butter, stirring constantly. Still stirring, add
milk slowly to form white sauce. Add cheese and stir until
melted. Spike with cayenne pepper, if desired. Serve over
leftover ratatouille.

LINGUINE WITH BROCCOLI AND ESCAROLE

Oil
1 garlic clove, chopped
½ head of broccoli, chopped and rinsed
Dried hot pepper, crumbled, or in flakes (optional)

12 mushrooms, sliced
¼ head of escarole, rinsed, drained and chopped
Soy sauce
½ pound cooked linguine

Heat oil in wok or skillet. Add garlic, broccoli and hot pepper and sauté over high heat, stirring, for a couple of minutes. Add mushrooms and stir thoroughly, less than 1 minute. Add the escarole, stir in, sprinkle with soy sauce, turn down heat, and cover. Let steam for one or two minutes. Toss with linguine and serve. *Serves 2.*

FETTUCCINE ALFREDO

A rich dish—quick, too—for family or company. Inspired by a letter from Barbara Chilcott, who makes a similar dish and reminded me of this standby from earlier days. It also has the merit of being relatively cheap, and healthier than the original Alfredo's noodles (he used heavy cream).

4 tablespoons butter
1 pound cooked fettuccine or other egg noodles
1 cup fresh grated Parmesan cheese

2 eggs, beaten
1 tablespoon lemon juice
½ cup yogurt
Fresh ground black pepper

Melt butter; toss with noodles and cheese over low heat. Beat eggs, lemon juice and yogurt together. Add to noodles, remove from heat and toss. Top with pepper. *Serves 4.*

LINGUINE WITH WHITE CLAM SAUCE

A quick and easy dish for an evening when you don't feel like fussing over dinner. It's also a pleasing dish for company, and if you want to be fancy about it, the deluxe version (recipe follows) can be fixed for little extra trouble.

2 tablespoons olive oil
1 can chopped clams
2 garlic cloves, minced
  Large pinch oregano
1 tablespoon fresh
  chopped parsley
2 tablespoons lemon
  juice

1 tablespoon yogurt
½ pound linguine,
  cooked
1 tablespoon butter
  Grated Parmesan
  cheese

Heat oil in a skillet. Drain clams and reserve liquid. Sauté garlic for 1 minute. Add clams, oregano and parsley. Sauté for 1 minute more. Add lemon juice and juice from clams. Simmer for a minute or two; stir in yogurt and remove from heat.

Toss linguine with butter over low heat. Serve topped with clam sauce and Parmesan cheese. *Serves 2.*

DELUXE LINGUINE WITH CLAM SAUCE

Garnished with fresh steamed clams, an elegant dish for company. Count on half a dozen clams per person. Scrub under cold water.

Prepare linguine recipe. While sauce is simmering, heat ½ cup water or beer in a heavy skillet. Steam clams open in skillet, covered. Serve linguine and sauce on a large platter with the clams arranged around the edges.

LINGUINE WITH BROCCOLI AND SCALLOPS

1 pound linguine
1 head broccoli
2 garlic cloves
6 tablespoons butter

1 pound bay scallops
Salt and pepper
Parmesan cheese

Cook linguine. Cut broccoli into florets and discard stem. Steam 2 minutes, rinse in cold water and set aside. Sauté garlic lightly in 4 tablespoons of the butter; add broccoli; stir to coat with butter, add scallops and cook 3 minutes. Rinse cooked linguine in cold water, return to heat and toss with 2 tablespoons butter, salt and pepper. Serve with scallops and broccoli spooned over the pasta and topped with grated Parmesan cheese.   *Serves 4.*

LINDA WINTERS'S BASIC TOMATO SAUCE WITH FENNEL

This basic sauce for spaghetti and other pasta dishes gets its special zest from the presence of the fennel, or finocchio, seeds beloved of Italian cooks.

½ cup chopped onion
2 garlic cloves,
   crushed
¼ cup olive oil

1–2 pound can Italian
   plum tomatoes,
   drained (reserve
   liquid)

1 tablespoon honey
1 tablespoon sea salt
1½ teaspoon dried basil
   leaves

4–6 fennel seeds, crushed
¼ teaspoon pepper
1 can tomato paste (see
   note)

Sauté onion and garlic in oil. Add half the tomatoes and the honey, salt, basil, fennel and pepper. Cook for a few minutes, then add the rest of the tomatoes, their juice and the tomato paste. *Enough for 1 pound of pasta.*

NOTE: Linda doesn't use the tomato paste, although it was called for in the recipe as she originally cooked it. Instead she drains off all the juice from the tomatoes and purées the tomatoes in a blender. The tomato paste makes a slightly thicker, saltier sauce. The version without paste may be used by people who are trying to watch their salt intake.

BASIC MARINARA SAUCE

This makes a simple and quick meal, served over pasta with cheese and complemented with a green salad. It is the heart of southern Italian cooking, by itself or as a base for the fish stews and sauces of a seafaring people. It is a key ingredient of pasta dishes like lasagne, ravioli, manicotti, shells and more, when served southern Italian–style. Use it in summer with fresh garden vegetables to make ratatouille.

1 medium onion,
   chopped
3 garlic cloves,
   chopped
1 tablespoon oregano
1 tablespoon basil
1 teaspoon thyme
½ bay leaf
1 tablespoon parsley
   and/or chopped
   celery leaves

¼ cup oil (preferably
   olive)
1 can (28 ounces) plum
   tomatoes, drained
   (reserve liquid)
½ small can tomato
   paste
1 teaspoon honey
   (optional)
Pinch of cayenne
   pepper

Sauté the onion, garlic and herbs in several tablespoons of the oil until transparent. Add the tomatoes and the balance of the oil if needed. Shred the tomatoes with a knife and fork as they cook over medium heat. Add the paste and the liquid from the tomatoes, and simmer about half an hour over low heat. Taste after a short while, and add honey if the sauce seems too acid. Add the cayenne pepper if you like it. Serve over spaghetti or other pasta with freshly grated cheese if available. *Serves 3–4.*

NOTES: Beverly Hanfield, who learned Italian cooking at her mother's side, was the one who educated me to the fact that good Italian sauce usually includes a sweetener of some kind and a taste of hot pepper.

Marinara sauces also frequently call for an anchovy fillet, and you may include it if you like the taste. I think the sauce is just as good without it. I don't use anchovies mainly because it's a nuisance to store the remainder of the can or tube in the refrigerator for the rare occasions when you will need it, and also because most people seem to dislike them.

The consistency of the sauce should be neither watery nor pasty. If it needs thickening, use more tomato paste. If it needs diluting, a little beer does the job and also takes the acid edge off the tomatoes. For added depth in flavor, you can add red wine.

LASAGNE FLORENTINE

A nonmeat lasagne using squash and spinach. This version is made without tomato sauce, but that may be added on the top of each layer if desired, using basic meatless marinara sauce.

1 pound fresh spinach, or 1 10-ounce package frozen, thawed and drained
2 tablespoons oil
3 garlic cloves
  Salt or soy sauce
1 medium onion, chopped
3 large squashes, 2 zucchini and 1 yellow, thinly sliced
½ pound lasagne noodles
1 pound ricotta cheese
¼ cup fresh chopped basil, if available, or ½ teaspoon dried
8 ounces mozzarella, grated
1 egg
1 cup plain yogurt
  Parmesan, Romano or other hard grating cheese

Set water for lasagne to boil. Set oven to preheat at 375 degrees. Wash and clean spinach, removing stems and discarding any spoiled leaves. Heat 1 tablespoon of the oil in a large skillet and sauté garlic. Add spinach and let it steam over low heat, covered, until limp. It may not all fit in at once; just keep adding it as the steaming process flattens it. When done, a matter of a minute or so, add a little salt or a little soy sauce, if desired. Set aside in a bowl. Wipe out pan, add remaining oil, and sauté onion; add squash and stir till slightly cooked and evenly covered with oil.

Cook the lasagne until almost done, 7–8 minutes; it helps to stir it after it gets limp in the pot, to prevent sticking. You may want to add a few drops of oil as well. When done, drain in a colander under cold water to rinse off starch and prevent sticking.

While the lasagne is cooking, mix the spinach and ricotta in a blender at low speed. If a blender isn't available and you are using fresh spinach, it can be more or less pulverized by grating it, but this is a tedious process. Add the basil.

Line bottom of a 9-by-12 greased baking pan with lasagne noodles. Cover with a layer of half the squash. Spread spinach mixture over the squash and sprinkle with half the mozzarella (any mild cheese will do in a pinch, e.g., longhorn, Cheddar). Add a layer of noodles. Spread with rest of the

squash. Beat egg into the yogurt and add remaining mozzarella. Pour over the squash and sprinkle with Parmesan.
Bake at 375 degrees until browned, 20 minutes or more.
Serve with plain sliced tomatoes on the side, or other raw
vegetables in season, as a garnish.   *Serves 6–8.*

CASSEROLES, OLD AND NEW

Give new life to old standbys like macaroni and cheese or tuna casserole by adding fresh vegetables from your supply of staples plus whatever is on hand—chopped celery, carrots and onions, even mushrooms, spinach or squash. For a summer casserole that's refreshingly light and inexpensive, try a Cheddar Squash Casserole.

MACARONI WITH CHEESE

2 cups cooked whole wheat macaroni, lightly salted
1 cup cottage cheese
½ cup grated Cheddar
1 rib celery, chopped
1 carrot, grated or chopped fine

1 medium onion, chopped
1 tablespoon melted butter
1 egg
2 cups milk
½ cup Deluxe Bread Crumbs (recipe follows)

In a greased baking dish, toss macaroni, cheeses, vegetables, and butter together. Beat egg and milk. Sprinkle macaroni mixture with bread crumbs and pour milk and egg over the casserole. Bake at 350 degrees for half an hour.   *Serves 2.*

DELUXE BREAD CRUMBS

2 slices whole wheat bread
1 small garlic clove
1 tablespoon Parmesan cheese

Fresh parsley, stems removed
1 teaspoon oregano (optional)

Break up bread. Combine with garlic, cheese and parsley (and oregano if you want an Italian flavor). Chop in blender. Store in refrigerator.

TUNA NOODLE CASSEROLE

An easy supper dish. Serve with Easy Green Salad (see Index).

3 cups cooked noodles
1 6-ounce can tuna, drained
6 fresh mushrooms, sliced
1 cup yogurt
½ small onion, chopped fine

½ carrot, cut into matchsticks
½ rib celery, chopped
3 tablespoons dry sherry (optional)
Bread crumbs

Toss all the ingredients except the bread crumbs together. Top the casserole with the crumbs, and bake at 350 degrees for 20–30 minutes.   *Serves 3–4.*

QUICK CHEDDAR-SQUASH CASSEROLE

Good as an entrée with a side dish of steamed carrots and cauliflower, or broccoli or brussels sprouts, or sliced tomatoes.

1 small zucchini, sliced
1 yellow squash, sliced
1½ cups cubes of stale bread, lightly toasted
½ cup grated Cheddar cheese

1 egg
1–2 cups milk
Parmesan cheese
Bread crumbs
Butter

Toss the squashes, the cubes of bread and the Cheddar cheese together in a large, lightly greased baking dish. Beat egg and milk together; there should be enough liquid to nearly cover the squash mixture. Sprinkle a mixture of Parmesan and bread crumbs on top and dot with butter. Bake half an hour at 350 degrees. *Makes 4 servings.*

CAROL'S EGGPLANT CASSEROLE

An invention from Carol Thompson's kitchen, using summer squashes and eggplant. Serve with salad or Fried Tomatoes (see Index) and rice or bread.

1 medium eggplant, cut into chunks and steamed 6 minutes	4 slices bread, cut into chunks and toasted
1 yellow squash, sliced	1 cup grated mild cheese
1 zucchini, sliced	Salt
1 large onion, chopped	Pinch of cayenne pepper
1 large green pepper, cut into chunks	2 eggs, beaten
Basil	1½ cups milk

In a greased baking dish, layer the vegetables, basil, bread, cheese, salt and cayenne pepper. Mix eggs and milk and pour over the casserole. Add a little more milk if mixture seems too dry. Bake at 350 degrees for about half an hour. *Makes 6 servings.*

EGGS AS AN ENTRÉE

Eggs can be the great standby on nights when you just don't feel like cooking, or eating much. They're good for leisurely lunches and brunches, too, or for weekend breakfasts. These recipes range from a refreshingly different scrambled egg to two easier-than-pie mock quiches.

BASIC OMELETS

The omelet (its Italian counterpart is the frittata) is a favorite dish in its native France for suppers as well as lunches. Its components are the outside envelope of cooked eggs, and the filling, which can include anything from chives to jelly. Here are instructions for cooking and filling the omelet, followed by suggestions for fillings. Make individual omelets or one big one that can be folded and sliced to serve several people. If you're feeding a crowd, you may want to make a Potato Frittata (see Index), which is easier to slice and serve.

2 eggs per person	Butter or oil
Salt and pepper	Filling

Beat the eggs with 1 tablespoon water per two eggs. Season with salt and pepper. Heat butter or oil over medium-high flame and add eggs. Form the omelet's characteristic layered effect by pulling cooked edges away from the pan's sides and letting uncooked eggs run out from center and under edges. You may help this process along by stirring the top of the omelet in a circular, flat motion with the fork and tipping the pan (sort of rocking it, really) back and forth to let the uncooked portion run to the edges. This all helps with the layering. When the uncooked surface of the omelet has no excess liquid egg on it, you are ready to fill it. Spread the filling on one half of the omelet and fold other half over, using spatula. Reduce heat and allow filling to heat for a minute or so, and serve.

FILLINGS

Some favorites are sliced or grated cheese, herbs, fresh raw or cooked vegetables, sour cream and chives. Try:

MUSHROOMS:
Fresh sliced mushrooms, with or without chopped onions or scallions, sautéed in a little butter. (Use same pan for eggs.)

SPANISH:
Chopped onions, green peppers and celery, sautéed in butter, with fresh chopped tomatoes and a pinch of thyme cooked briefly until tomatoes disintegrate.

FINES HERBES:
French for fresh chopped parsley, basil and thyme (or your favorite combination), sautéed briefly with chives or scallions.

LEFTOVERS:
Just a reminder, as they surely need no explaining. Cooked vegetables, leftover stir-fry with or without rice, anything you think sounds good with perhaps a handful of grated cheese thrown in. The dark green vegetables—broccoli, spinach, escarole—go especially well with eggs and cheese.

SPINACH:
Fresh spinach cleaned and sautéed briefly with onions, garlic or mushrooms. Goes well with a sour cream substitute—cottage cheese mixed with yogurt.

CHEESE:
If you're using it, leave the omelet on the heat long enough to melt the cheese. Can be combined with vegetables of any kind.

POTATO FRITTATA

A hearty meal, with a side dish of sliced tomatoes or salad.

Oil	6 eggs
4–6 new potatoes, sliced thin	Salt and pepper
1 medium onion, chopped	

Heat oil, with some butter if desired, over medium-high flame. Add potatoes and onions, allow to brown, and turn. Allow to brown on other side. If potatoes are not yet tender, add a little water and turn down heat. Beat eggs with 2 tablespoons water. Sprinkle potatoes with salt and pepper, adding a dash of cayenne if desired. Pour eggs over potatoes. When underside of frittata is firm, slide it onto a plate, invert pan over plate, and turn right side up. Return pan to heat and let frittata finish cooking. Cut in quarters.   *Makes 4 servings.*

NOTE: Vary, using any firm vegetable. Softer fillings may be used by adding them to the eggs before cooking.

YOGURT SCRAMBLED EGGS

A deliciously tender and fluffy version of an old favorite. Serve with Fried Tomatoes (see Index).

6 eggs	1 tablespoon butter
3 tablespoons yogurt	Salt and pepper

Beat the eggs with the yogurt. Melt the butter over medium-high heat. Add the eggs and cook, stirring gently with a wooden spoon and scraping the sides and bottom of the pan to allow large curds to form. When the eggs are done but not dry, season with salt and pepper and serve. The yogurt helps keep this dish moist.　*Serves 3.*

POACHED EGGS WITH CHEESE SAUCE

A good brunch or light supper. Serve with sliced tomatoes or a salad.

2–3　cups Cheese Sauce 　　(recipe follows)
　8　eggs

1　teaspoon vinegar
4　English muffins, split

Make the Cheese Sauce. Then poach the eggs in a large skillet full of gently boiling water to which 1 teaspoon of vinegar has been added to help keep the egg yolks intact. While they are poaching, toast the muffins—or make toast if you prefer. Remove eggs from pan with a slotted spoon or spatula, and serve on muffins. Top with sauce.　*Serves 4.*

CHEESE SAUCE

This is a white sauce with cheese in it. Use it for vegetables or eggs, or with your pasta primavera if you like.

2　cups milk
2　tablespoons butter
2　tablespoons flour

1　cup grated cheese
Dash of cayenne 　pepper

Heat milk. Melt butter; stir flour into butter. Add hot milk, stirring constantly to yield a white sauce that is thickened but not pasty. Thin if necessary with hot water or milk. Add cheese and stir over low heat to melt. Add cayenne, if desired.

JEANNE'S UNHURRIED BRUNCH

An attractive egg-and-tomato meal that can be served in individual baking dishes if you have them.

6 cherry tomatoes per person	Parmesan cheese
Butter	1–2 eggs per person
Bread crumbs	Salt and pepper
	Thyme

Halve the tomatoes and arrange around baking dishes, leaving space in the center. Put a pat of butter in center and cook under broiler 1–2 minutes, until tomatoes look tender. Turn oven to 350 degrees and remove dishes.

Cover the tomatoes and center of dishes with bread crumbs and Parmesan cheese. Break 1 or 2 eggs into each dish and sprinkle with salt, pepper and a little thyme. Cook until eggs are done, about 2 minutes.

NOTE: Jeanne Eichelberger, who devised this meal, adds that if no cherry tomatoes are available tomato wedges work just as well. We have found that if you don't have individual baking dishes a larger dish or greased pie pan does just as well, though extricating the eggs without breakage can be tricky. Gently separate them with a spatula to serve.

TUNA QUICHE CASSEROLE

A delicious main dish with an understated crust. Serve with a green salad or with steamed vegetables.

THE FILLING:
2 cans (6½ ounces each) tuna, drained
½ cup shredded Cheddar cheese
¼ cup chopped onion
¼ cup chopped celery
¼ cup chopped almonds
2 tablespoons lemon juice
1 egg
½ teaspoon salt
¼ teaspoon pepper

THE DOUGH:
2 cups flour
1 tablespoon baking powder
⅔ cup milk
¼ cup yogurt
1 egg yolk, beaten

Mix ingredients for filling. Mix dough, excepting egg yolk, and spread half of it in an 8-inch baking pan. Top with filling. Spread rest of dough on top of filling and brush with egg yolk. Bake at 400 degrees for 25–30 minutes. *Makes 6–8 servings.*

GARDEN VEGETABLE PIE

This is quicker and easier than making a quiche and achieves the same result: a nice, custardy entrée that goes well with a simple green salad for dinner. This is Jeanne Eichelberger's version.

1½ cups milk
½ cup flour
2–3 eggs
1 teaspoon salt
½ teaspoon pepper
2 cups broccoli, cauliflower or squash, chopped
½ cup chopped onions
½ cup chopped green peppers
1 cup shredded Cheddar cheese (about 4 ounces)

Blend milk, flour, eggs, salt and pepper. Stir in rest of ingredients and pour into a 9- or 10-inch casserole dish. Bake 35–40 minutes in a 400-degree oven. *Makes 4 servings.*

RICE DISHES

If you haven't made rice the centerpiece of a meal, stir-fry is a good place to start, as are curries. Both can be dressed up for company with side dishes, with curries looking especially festive with all their condiments. Both can be made with or without meat or poultry or fish, depending on what strategy you are pursuing. In any case, with the vegetables in stir-fry and the sauce for curry, you will be extending the non-meat elements of the dish and greatly reducing the amount of animal protein you use. This is a strategy that can be applied to all dishes using animal protein, of course. You are the one controlling the balance of the ingredients in any dish, and it is good to remember that most recipes can be varied a great deal to suit the user without any bad results.

The recipes for stir-fry and curry include one with chicken and one with shrimp, but these are interchangeable with any kind of fish or fowl prepared in bite-size pieces, or with no animal flesh, but just vegetables and nuts.

STIR-FRIED VEGETABLES

This can be a meal in itself, or can be amplified by adding chicken or shrimp, as given below. I even use it as a recipe that doubles for meat eaters and non-meat eaters, by dividing the vegetables after they're done and quickly stir-frying some sliced steak to add to the meat eaters' portions. So if you have no objection to cooking meat for others, that's an option, too. The basic vegetables for this are carrots, onions and celery, plus whatever else is handy, including some nuts. This version suggests other vegetables; use what you have.

5 large mushrooms
1 carrot
1 small onion
1 rib celery, with leaves
½ green pepper
  Broccoli or cauliflower
    florets
  Handful of thinly
    sliced cabbage
  Handful of bean
    sprouts

¼ eggplant or ½
    zucchini squash,
    sliced and cut into
    matchsticks
  Small handful of
    walnuts
1 tablespoon oil
1 teaspoon sesame seeds
2 teaspoons tamari
    sauce

Slice all the vegetables and chop nuts. They may be sliced in thin rounds (straight for the mushrooms, diagonal for the carrot), or cut in half moons (onions) or further sliced into matchsticks (squash), or any combination of these.

Heat the oil in a wok or large skillet. Add the vegetables, starting with the sturdier ones that will take longer to cook—carrot, onion, broccoli, pepper—then the less sturdy, including celery and eggplant, plus the nuts and seeds. Last are the delicate squash and mushrooms, and then any leafy vegetables. Stir constantly.

When the last vegetables are just coated with oil, add tamari and cover. Cook on reduced heat for just a minute or so, not long enough to make the vegetables soggy. Serve over rice.   *Makes 3–4 servings.*

WITH CHICKEN, SHRIMP OR OTHER MEAT:

Just before any leafy vegetables, but after everything else, scrape the vegetables aside, add a bit more oil, and quickly sauté the meat (which should be sliced in advance like everything else) or shrimp. Then proceed with tamari and finish.

Shrimp should be cleaned in advance, but can be cooked whole.

For chicken, use ½ breast for two people. Bone it by cutting the meat free where it joins the breastbone and pulling it off the rib bones.

Don't waste the bones with shreds of meat attached. Put

them right into enough water to cover and boil until bones are clean. Then use the broth with bits of meat for a quick Chicken Corn Chowder, or freeze in ice trays and then store in a plastic bag in the freezer for instant chicken broth.

HOT AND SPICY:
To achieve a mildly spicy effect, add chopped fresh ginger or dried ginger with the sturdy vegetables. For a hot Szechuan stir-fry, add fresh or dried peppers—jalapeño or any other hot red or green peppers—sliced or crumbled, with the sturdy vegetables.

WITH TOFU:
Stir-fry can be an easy introduction for the family to the Oriental bean curd cake, tofu. If you haven't already experimented with it in your cooking, try it this way. Dice about a quarter of a tofu cake and add it to the hot oil with the sturdy vegetables. It will turn golden brown and crispy as your stir-fry progresses.

SIMPLE RICE AND BEANS

A good, easy supper. Serve with Taco Salad (see Index).

2 cups brown rice	1 teaspoon basil
1 onion, chopped	1 can (10 or 12 ounces)
½ green pepper, chopped	kidney beans or other beans
1 garlic clove, diced	2 tablespoons tamari
Pinch of salt	Chopped scallions

Cook rice, onion, pepper, garlic, salt and basil in 3 cups water. When all liquid is absorbed, stir in the beans, with liquid, and tamari, and simmer an additional 10 minutes. Garnish with chopped scallions.   *Serves 3–4.*

BASIC CURRY SAUCE

This is like a white sauce to which cooked vegetables or chicken or shrimp can be added. If you are adding raw vegetables or flesh food, you should put them in with the onions and curry powder, before the liquid and the yogurt.

A curry is traditionally served with rice and garnishes of chutney, raisins, nuts, shredded coconut, chopped onions and/or chopped hardcooked egg. Side dishes often include *dal*—cooked lentils or dried split peas—and cooked dark greens, such as collards or kale.

1 medium onion,
  chopped
1 garlic clove, chopped
  Oil
2 tablespoons Basic
  Curry Powder (see
  Index)

1 cup cooked or raw
  vegetables, chicken
  or fish
3 tablespoons yogurt

Sauté onion and garlic in oil. Add curry powder (and raw ingredients, if any) and sauté briefly. Add 2 cups water or broth and simmer 5 minutes on low heat. Add cooked ingredients and simmer 5 minutes more. Remove from heat and stir in yogurt. Serve with rice and garnishes. *Enough for 3–4 servings.*

NOTE: Needless to say, this is a handy way of dispatching leftover vegetables and chicken. In fact, that may be how it originated. Indian restaurants seldom serve this curry, which may mean that it is deemed unworthy fare for dining out.

SIDE VEGETABLES

For times when you have the time and energy to make more than a one-dish meal, or when you want a more ample dinner, put together a side dish from staple vegetables that keep well, or from seasonal vegetables. You'll find that vegetables cook in just minutes in a steamer—be careful not to overcook them. Sautéing or stir-frying requires your attention. If you're cooking another dish that needs constant attention, like pan-poached fish, you'll want to scrub and otherwise prepare the vegetables for cooking before starting the other dish.

ARTICHOKES

Seasonal, winter and spring. An elegant dish for company. Cut off the stem and remove small leaves at base. If desired, trim off sharp points of leaves. Boil in salted water with basil or thyme added for about 40 minutes. Allow 1 small artichoke per person. Serve with melted butter and lemon juice for dipping the leaves, the soft underside of which is then scraped off with the teeth. When the artichoke has been eaten down to the softest leaves and the fine hairlike leaves exposed, this part is cut off and the "heart" eaten with knife and fork.

To make a quick hollandaise for 4, combine ½ cup hot melted butter with juice of ½ lemon and blend with 3 egg yolks.

ASPARAGUS VINAIGRETTE

Seasonal, available in spring. Rinse thoroughly and tie loosely in a bundle top and bottom, so that the bunch may support itself during cooking. Steam standing up in a tall stockpot with a lid. If desired, shorten asparagus by breaking off the stalks where they bend most easily—usually just above the white part—since the lower stems won't be eaten because of toughness. If you don't have a tall pot, asparagus may be steamed in a regular steamer or colander, or even cooked by boiling 3–5 minutes. The stand-up method is preferred as the one that tenderizes the stalk most evenly.

Toss the cooked asparagus gently in Basic Vinaigrette Dressing (see Index) and serve warm. Asparagus may also be served plain, with a little butter and lemon. One bunch serves 4. Goes well with fish and chicken dishes.

BROCCOLI, CARROTS AND ONIONS

A nice bright dish that requires little fuss. Scrub carrots, rinse broccoli and peel onions, allowing 1 carrot, ¼ head broccoli and 1 small onion per person. Cut carrots and onions into bite-size pieces; remove broccoli leaves, cutting broccoli florets and upper stems into bite-size pieces. Steam carrots and onions until almost tender, 5–7 minutes; add broccoli and steam 2–3 minutes more, until barely tender. Serve at once, tossed with a little butter, salt and pepper. Good with all chicken and fish dishes, casseroles and omelets.

CABBAGE-CARROT STIR-FRY

The staple cabbage, carrots and onions can be thrown together to expand or brighten up a meal. With a handful of broken nut meats, this also makes a great emergency one-dish meal over rice. Thinly slice 1 carrot and ½ onion per person; slice and set aside about a handful of cabbage shreds per person. Sauté the carrots and onions in a very little oil over high heat until well done, even a little scorched. Turn down heat, add cabbage, and toss together. Add 1 teaspoon tamari sauce per person, cover, and cook 1 minute. Serve over rice or on the side. Good with any fish or chicken dish, or as a meal in itself.

CINNAMON CARROTS

Steam carrots, scrubbed and cut into quarters, until tender. Allow 1 carrot per serving. Toss cooked carrots in melted butter (about 2 teaspoons per serving) to which cinnamon (1 large pinch per serving) and honey (½ teaspoon per serving) have been added. Stir over low heat until carrots are nicely coated. Especially nice with plain chicken dishes.

ITALIAN GREEN BEANS

Rinse and pinch off ends of 1 pound beans, leaving otherwise whole unless they're very long. A pound will serve about 6 people. Steam until tender, 5–10 minutes, with a large pinch of rosemary and a large clove of garlic, sliced thin. Then sauté briefly in a very little olive oil. Garnish with lemon juice and/or sliced almonds.

SNOW PEAS AND MUSHROOMS

Sauté ½ pound cleaned mushrooms in 4 tablespoons butter or light oil. Add a pinch of ginger. Add 1 pound snow peas, rinsed and cleaned (pinch off ends of pods and pull "strings," if any) and sauté, stirring, 3–4 minutes. Good with any dish, and nice for company.   *Serves 4.*

SUMMER SQUASHES

Cut into quarters and steam 1 zucchini or yellow squash per person. Season with butter or just salt and pepper. Good with any of the richer dishes.

WINTER SQUASHES

Scrub, dry and bake at 350 degrees an acorn or any other winter squash, until easily pierced with a fork, 15–20 minutes. Split open and scrape out seeds and strings. Add a small pat of butter and a dash of cinnamon to the cavity of each squash and return to oven for 5 minutes or so. The butternut squash won't need butter. One squash serves 2. Especially good with the meatier dishes and the Oriental entrées.

YAMS

Prick with a fork and bake at 350 degrees until tender, about 15 minutes. This very underrated tuber is a great side dish for any fish or chicken dish, or any dish made with rice or other whole grains.

LEFTOVERS VINAIGRETTE

Any steamed vegetable can be marinated overnight and served as a salad, or taken to work for lunch. Toss the marinated vegetables together with leftover pasta or rice for a heartier salad.

STEAMED VEGETABLES AS A SIDE DISH

Apart from cutting them up, steamed vegetables require virtually no preparation. Eat them as often as you can. They offer these advantages:

■ They contain no fat, sugar or salt unless you add it.
■ They add bulk to your diet and bright colors to your plate.
■ Added to casserole entrées, they make a hearty meal that anyone can enjoy.
■ They are rich in essential vitamins and minerals. And if you can include dark green vegetables, they offer the chlorophyll that Oriental healers believe builds stronger blood. Those dark green vegetables, in any case, are chock-full of vitamin A, which people who work inside under artificial light need.

Common sense and trial and error are a great team in cooking. You'll know what size carrot chunk cooks quickly, but not too quickly, in your steamer after you've tried it. In general, don't peel vegetables unless their skins are hard, tough, or brittle. Just scrub them well with a brush reserved for that purpose. Be suspicious of tough-looking stems; they probably are, and should be split (broccoli) or scored (brussels sprouts). The best way to tell if a vegetable is done is to poke it quickly with a sharp fork. You'll recognize the texture you like.

Try combinations of vegetables in season—carrots and string beans, carrots and broccoli, yellow and green squash, brussels sprouts and onions. Season them with lemon juice and a little salt and pepper just before serving. Add herbs to the cooking water for a subtle flavor.

INDIAN SIDE DISHES

Good with curries and other Eastern dishes, these are frequently found as side dishes in Indian restaurants. They are all easy to make.

CUCUMBER SALAD

2 cucumbers, sliced thin	½ cup yogurt
1 onion, chopped	1 tablespoon fresh or
Salt	dried crushed mint
Juice of 1 lemon	leaves

Toss ingredients together and chill for an hour or more.

For a drier mixture, salt the cucumbers and toss the other ingredients together separately. Let the cucumbers stand for half an hour; chill the yogurt mixture. Drain the cucumbers, add the yogurt mixture, and chill for half an hour. *Makes 4 servings.*

DAL

As a side dish, it is mild. It can also be made with curry powder and a spice called asafetida (just a pinch, it's strong) for a spicier main dish.

1 small onion, chopped	1 cup lentils or split
½ carrot, chopped fine	peas
1 tablespoon oil	

Sauté onion and carrot in the oil. Add 2 cups water and lentils or peas. Cook until tender. *Serves 2.*

COOKED GREENS

1 garlic clove	1 tablespoon tamari
1 teaspoon oil	1 tablespoon lemon
½ pound greens	juice
(escarole, spinach,	
collards, or	
dandelion greens,	
for example)	

Sauté garlic in oil. Add greens and cook until wilted. Add tamari and lemon juice and toss over heat for half a minute. *Serves 2.*

FRIED TOMATOES

An excellent side dish with eggs for brunch, lunch and even supper. Fried tomatoes are an old favorite in our family, where they have been known to make a whole meal in themselves, eaten with brown bread and butter and a large pot of tea. They're good cold, too.

Corn meal for	1 tomato per person
dredging	Oil
Salt and pepper	

Mix corn meal, salt and pepper on a large plate. Slice the tomatoes and dredge to cover both sides with the corn meal mixture. Fry in oil over medium-high heat, preferably in a heavy skillet, turning tomatoes once to brown on both sides.

NOTE: Some people use flour for fried tomatoes. The corn meal is a Southern addition, and we like its texture and flavor better than the flour. But you can use either, or a mixture. A tablespoon or so of wheat germ or Parmesan cheese is a welcome addition, too.

WHAT ABOUT LUNCH?

Everyone can exercise creativity and control in making sandwiches. There are too many possibilities to be catalogued, but you may want to keep a certain amount of basic salad mix on hand, augmenting it with perishables like sliced tomato, avocado, onion or whatever.

Good basics are egg salad and tuna salad made with yogurt or cottage cheese to eliminate some of the mayonnaise (or all, for those on diets). Jazz up sandwiches like cheese or tuna by adding shredded carrots as well as lettuce; use other greens, too. Lots of people know about peanut butter and banana sandwiches, but I like peanut butter with sliced apple.

If you have leftover soup, carry it along in a Thermos. Cold stir-fry and rice is also quite a fine lunch, if there's any of that left over. Again, keep it simple and it will be easier to keep it all working smoothly. Lunch doesn't need to be an elaborate meal, and you don't need a recipe to make a cheese sandwich.

KEEP BREAKFAST SIMPLE, TOO

I have suggested that you spare the eggs for lunch and dinner dishes, but if breakfast is your main meal, by all means get your animal protein there.

This may be the case especially on weekends, when people enjoy a leisurely meal with family or friends before going out for a day's activities. For those occasions, pancakes can be whipped up quickly and make everybody happy, especially if there's fresh fruit to go on top.

For everyday breakfasts, cereal is the best mainstay. And don't forget the fruit—for bulk, vitamins, minerals and carbohydrate energy.

EASY PANCAKES

If you have grown up using a prepared pancake mix, you may know its proportions by heart—1 cup mix, 1 cup milk, 1 egg, 1 tablespoon oil. If you look at my recipe here, you'll see I have pretty much the same proportions. That's because my dry ingredients are exactly what you'd find in a dry mix.

You can make your own "prepared" mix in limited quantities if you have a reasonably cool, dry place to put it. The refrigerator isn't too good for the salt and baking powder, and you don't want the flour to sit too long in a hot place because of rancidity. Something in between is good. Your "prepared" mix would consist of just the dry ingredients.

DRY INGREDIENTS:
- 1 cup unbleached flour
- 2 teaspoons baking powder
- 1 teaspoon salt

WET INGREDIENTS:

| 1 cup milk | 1 tablespoon oil |
| 1 egg | |

Mix the dry ingredients, pressing any lumps out of the flour. Beat the wet ingredients and add to the dry, mixing until the batter is wet through. Don't worry about getting all the lumps out of the batter, though you can press out the large ones.

Heat a little butter or oil in a heavy iron skillet; wipe most of it out with a paper towel, which you set aside. When the skillet is hot enough that a drop of water will dance on it, ladle in enough batter to make one large cake, and tip the pan so that it spreads evenly and is not too thick. Cook on first side until top surface is covered with bubbles; turn, cook briefly and remove to a warm plate. If desired, put a thin pat of butter on the cake to melt as you start the next one.

If the skillet starts to smoke, lift it up off the heat periodically while you continue cooking, or turn the heat down. If you have a gas stove, you can play with the heat until you get it right. Grease the skillet as needed by wiping with the greasy paper towel. *Serves 2 hungry people.*

NOTES: If you prefer to make small cakes, go right ahead. I like to make a tall stack of big cakes and then cut them into as many parts as there are people.

Your batter consistency is as important as getting the heat right. Don't hesitate to add more liquid—milk or water—to make a batter that runs smoothly off the spoon but is not runny. If the cakes don't bubble in cooking, you need more baking powder; just stir it into the batter. If the batter in the bowl is very bubbly, you have too much baking powder; add a little more flour and liquid.

Much of this depends on the flour. Get to know the character of your brand of flour. Again, unbleached may require more liquid and perhaps more baking powder than bleached. I have had good results with 2 teaspoons of baking powder, but often I find I have to add more liquid after starting with the basic measure of 1 cup. The batter may be stored for several days in the refrigerator. Stir and add liquid if needed before using.

DELUXE PANCAKE MIX

DRY INGREDIENTS:

1 cup unbleached flour
¼ cup corn meal
2 tablespoons wheat germ

2 tablespoons bran
1 teaspoon salt
1 tablespoon baking powder

WET INGREDIENTS:

2 eggs
1 cup milk (or more)
1 tablespoon oil

Water as needed to thin batter

Prepare as for Easy Pancakes (see Index). For another variation, substitute ¼ cup rolled oats that have been run through the blender for the corn meal.

The addition of the other grains to the mixture makes a crisp, glossy pancake.

TOPPINGS:

Maple syrup, honey, cooked fruit and yogurt are all good. Cooked fruit is a good addition to syrup because it dilutes the sugar content of the topping.

One late spring morning before any of the season's fruit had come in, I hauled out a package of blueberries frozen last summer and added a handful still frozen to the batter. Another handful went into a saucepan with a tablespoon of honey, to thaw over a low flame, making a delicious and less-sweet topping. It was a real treat. Apples, peaches and various berries are good, too.

BASIC GRANOLA

Make it in large batches in the oven—be sure to get it thoroughly dry, which requires periodic stirring so that it doesn't burn at the same time. It has to be quite dry if you are going to store it on the shelf, or it will become moldy. This is just a matter of a little patience, but you'll definitely know when it's dry because it will go from soggy to crunchy. A good dish to bake when you're home on an evening just puttering around, and keep it on hand for "instant" breakfasts.

1 cup apple juice	¼ cup sesame, sunflower
¼ cup honey	or pumpkin seeds
¼ cup oil	1 tablespoon cinnamon
1 teaspoon vanilla	1 teaspoon nutmeg
7 cups rolled oats	1 cup raisins
½ cup chopped walnuts	

Heat the apple juice, honey, oil and vanilla to boiling and remove from heat. Stir in the oats to moisten thoroughly. Mix in the nuts, seeds, cinnamon and nutmeg. Do not add the raisins yet. Bake the mixture in a 325-degree oven until it is crisp and dry, stirring frequently. Remove from oven, add raisins, and allow to cool. Store in airtight jars in a cool, dark place.

NOTES: If you add the raisins before baking, they'll burn or get hard. Or both.

If you want a crispier and easier-to-handle product, omit the juice and increase the amount of honey by ¼ cup, or add ¼ cup maple syrup. The fruit juice—and any mild juice will do, by the way—is to sweeten the granola without having to use so much honey.

PARTY FOODS

Simplicity is the key here, too. A party should not lead to despair on the part of the host. A good dip for raw vegetables can be made a day or so in advance; time must be left right before the party to slice the vegetables so they don't get stale, but they can be cleaned in advance. Good quality cheeses and crackers can be set out where people can help themselves. Stuffed eggs are offered with any easy method for stuffing them in quantity. For fancier fare, steamed shellfish can be prepared by cleaning in advance, steaming while the party is in progress, and letting guests help themselves. And a bowl of cleaned fruit set out will find its audience as the party wears on.

GARLIC-PARSLEY DIP

A simple dip for parties. Serve with sliced raw vegetables.

8 ounces small-curd cottage cheese	2 tablespoons lemon juice
4 tablespoons chopped fresh parsley	1 teaspoon tamari Yogurt
2 garlic cloves, chopped	

Blend cottage cheese with parsley and garlic. Season with lemon juice and tamari. Stir in a little yogurt for a creamier texture.

NOTE: Use basil instead of parsley if desired.

STUFFED EGGS À LA BILL COYLE

One dark New Year's Eve when about fifty guests were impending, it was Coyle who introduced to our house the technique of stuffing lots of eggs in a hurry. We recommend it if you are thinking of having them as hors d'oeuvres.

2 dozen eggs, hard-boiled	1 tablespoon Dijon mustard
¼ cup mayonnaise	Salt and pepper
2 tablespoons yogurt	
1 tablespoon lemon juice	

Mix the egg yolks with the mayonnaise, yogurt, lemon juice and mustard. Add salt and pepper if needed. Add more mayonnaise or yogurt if needed for a moist filling.

To stuff the eggs, take a clean, fairly sturdy plastic bag, and cut off the corner of one side to form a small hole. Put the filling into the bag and force it into the centers of the whites, pastry tube-style. Garnish with paprika or parsley if desired.

Added advantage: The plastic bag can be discarded when you're done, leaving one less thing to clean up.

ABOUT BAKING

Quick breads and other baked goods that don't require yeast are a good place to start if you are learning baking. They are quick, easy, and give you a feel for handling things made with flour, which definitely has a personality.

If you are an experienced baker, the following will simply provide a handy point of reference as basic recipes. If you are a beginner, they provide a point of departure.

Among non-yeast baked goods there are those that require handling and those that don't. The latter include muffins, some loaf breads, and pancakes, all made from batter that is stirred together and then cooked.

Doughs that require handling include biscuits and pie crust. Biscuits are easier because they are less unwieldy—pie crust being thinner and larger. From pie crust it is a short logical step to homemade noodles. Yeast breads, once you have the feel of the yeast, are actually easier.

The advantage of doing your own baking whenever practical is that you can control the quantity and quality of the ingredients; and, of course, you have the satisfaction of eating the biscuits fresh out of the oven.

With recipes for baked goods from cookbooks, I often find that the proportions of ingredients have to be adjusted. This may be because of the unbleached flour soaking up more liquid, or it may have to do with other factors, such as altitude and humidity. Flour is a plastic substance that acts differently in different circumstances. Let your dough be your guide. In batters, the ingredients should be mixed only enough to distribute the liquid ingredients evenly through the dry ingredients, and get rid of any outstanding lumps. In muffins, for instance, it is important not to mix too thoroughly, as this makes the muffins heavy.

In biscuit and pie dough, the fat (butter, margarine, Crisco) is cut into the dry ingredients first, using a pastry blender, or a knife and fork, or two knives against each other to break up the fat until the flour has a consistency usually described as being like corn meal. The remaining lumps of fat are described as being no larger than small peas. Then the liquids are added quickly and mixed in. The dough must be wet enough to stick together, but dry enough so that a thin dusting of flour on the rolling surface will make the dough manageable, whether you're using your hands or a rolling pin.

So the first thing to remember is that the proportions of ingredients in a baking recipe represent an educated suggestion at best. The second thing to remember is that you *will* recognize manageable dough, even if you've never handled it before. Unmanageable dough either falls to pieces (too dry) or, in the words of one veteran noodle maker, "sticks irrevocably to everything." (Then it's too wet.) The third thing to remember is that refined flour is not as heavy as whole wheat or even unbleached flour, and these better flours will give you a more substantial product than what you buy in a store. Your baked goods will by no means be leaden, but they may be heavier, moister, and richer than what you've been used to.

Quick breads, with their reliance on baking powder, baking soda, eggs and fat as leavening agents, are less digestible and so not as good for you as yeast breads, which in turn are not as good as sourdough and unyeasted breads. But they are an important introduction to the ways of flour, and they bridge the gap between reliance on commercial products and greater expertise in home baking. And they taste terrific.

Remember to store flour in the refrigerator in large clear plastic containers or glass jars, preferably with a tight-fitting lid. Label the containers for easy reference. Or with a flour you will be using often, simply slip the bag of flour inside a plastic bag. This helps keep the flour dry in the refrigerator and prevents spills in the refrigerator or on your counters. Whatever spills in handling is caught inside the bag.

All kinds of quick breads are just that; most take an hour or less to fix from start to finish. They include loaf breads, biscuits, muffins, corn bread and even pancakes. Like salad with real dressing, like vegetables that are fresh, they are more satisfying than their mass-produced counterparts. And while it helps in learning to make yeast breads to have someone walk you through it the first time, quick breads get their rise from soda and/or baking powder with minimal help from you, and you can follow a recipe and expect to have palatable results.

If you elect to make quick breads using unbleached flour and/or whole grain flours, you must not be alarmed if they turn out heavier than the commercial breads, even the "whole grain" commercial breads. You'll quickly come to appreciate the heavier homemade breads over their commercial counterparts, so don't conclude you've made a mistake. Also, if you're switching from bleached flour to unbleached or whole grain, you may notice these soak up more liquid than bleached, and you'll have to adjust recipes accordingly. The amount of baking powder or soda may be increased if rising seems to be a problem; you can always play with the rising agent in baking as one of the variables that also include the liquid and the dry ingredients. The recipes that follow presume unbleached flour and a reduced amount of sweeteners.

BASIC BISCUITS

Flaky, moist and tender, biscuits are a staple of old-fashioned Southern hospitality, and they do a lot for a simple meal. They take about 20 minutes once you are familiar with the recipe, and can make numbers of people very happy for hours. Serve them to make a simple soup or stew into a real meal. They don't taste as good the next day, but can be toasted and served with preserves for dessert or breakfast.

2 cups all-purpose
    unbleached flour,
    sifted
1 tablespoon baking
    powder

1 teaspoon salt
4 tablespoons butter
⅔ cup milk

In a large mixing bowl, combine flour, baking powder and salt and stir well. Cut in the butter with a knife and fork, or two knives, or a pastry blender, until flour has the texture of coarse corn meal and remaining lumps of butter are the size of small peas.

Make a well in the flour, and add the milk. Stir quickly into flour to form a moist dough.

Turn dough onto a well-floured board. Sift a little flour onto dough and knead briefly, 8–10 times. Pat dough into a thick flat slab and roll out to thickness of about ¾ of an inch. If the rolling pin sticks, dust it or the dough with flour.

Cut out biscuits with a biscuit cutter or the end of a small can (soup can, juice can, baking powder can) from which both ends have been removed. Press firmly; do not twist the cutter. Lay the biscuits on an ungreased cookie sheet and prick each one with a fork. Bake at 450 degrees for 10–12 minutes, until golden.   *Makes 12 large or 24 small biscuits.*

NOTES: A warming basket is a handy thing to have if you serve much hot bread. It also works for baked potatoes and sweet potatoes.

You can buy or make a warming basket. It consists of a stout basket four to six inches deep; a napkin or dish towel; and a flat stone or square of marble large enough to fill the bottom of the basket.

While the biscuits are baking, the stone is heated in the oven. It is set in the basket when the biscuits come out of the oven, and the biscuits, folded in the napkin, go on top of it. Keeps them warm throughout the meal. (In a pinch, a small pie plate of pebbles will do the trick, though it's less convenient.)

"Buttermilk" Yogurt Biscuits

These incredibly tender biscuits were the result of a night when there wasn't any baking powder in the house. That fine old reference book *The Joy of Cooking* confirmed that baking soda could be used if there was a soured milk product available to provide the acid to interact with the soda. There was. It was, of course, the staple plain yogurt.

For the milk in the Basic Biscuits recipe (see Index), substitute ½ cup yogurt and ½ cup milk. For the baking powder, substitute ⅓ teaspoon (*not* tablespoon) baking soda. Proceed as for the basic recipe. You may find you prefer these to the regular biscuits. Of course you may use buttermilk instead of both milk and yogurt—⅔ to 1 cup buttermilk.

Bran Muffins

A good addition to breakfast, if cereal isn't enough.

1 cup whole wheat flour, sifted	1 cup milk
1 cup bran	1 tablespoon melted butter or oil
1 tablespoon baking powder	1 egg, beaten
Pinch of salt	3 tablespoons honey
½ cup broken nut meats, or ¼ cup raisins	2 tablespoons molasses

Mix dry ingredients together. Mix wet ingredients, add to dry, and mix quickly to moisten batter, which should drop readily off a spoon. If necessary, add more milk, or add yogurt or buttermilk, to moisten.

Pour batter into muffin tins, filling each about ¾ full. Bake at 375 degrees for 20–30 minutes. Serve hot. *Makes one dozen.*

NOTE: Leftover muffins can be reheated by grilling them on a buttered skillet. Split muffins, grill and serve.

BASIC CORN BREAD

This is delicious with soups, and is quick and easy. Good for breakfast too! To get that good gritty texture and corny taste that go with Southern corn bread, use yellow corn meal, preferably stone or water ground, and a heavy pan (an iron skillet works fine) that has been greased and set in the oven while you're making the batter. This is essential—the batter must go into a hot pan—to get the texture right. The same goes for muffin tins, if you want to use the recipe for muffins.

¾ cup flour, sifted	1 cup milk
1 tablespoon baking powder	1 tablespoon honey
Pinch of salt	1 egg
1¼ cups yellow corn meal	3 tablespoons melted butter

Mix the dry ingredients and the wet ingredients separately. Combine, stirring a few times to moisten batter thoroughly. Pour batter into hot skillet, and bake for about 25 minutes in a 425-degree oven. *Makes 8 servings.*

NOTES: If you're using an iron skillet, baking time may be less. Keep an eye on the bread.

If the corn bread seems too gritty, you can adjust the texture next time by heating the milk and letting the corn meal soak in it while you mix the other dry and wet ingredients, then add milk with corn meal last and stir in.

BASIC NUT BREAD

This recipe is adapted from Dolores Casella's *A World of Breads*, given to me years ago by Esten Goolrick. It was the book out of which I learned to bake 12 loaves of bread once a week for a co-op dormitory dining room full of hungry people. I recommend it as a peerless book for bakers of all levels, from expert to totally ignorant.

¾ cup honey	5 cups unbleached flour
1 tablespoon molasses	1 teaspoon salt
½ cup melted butter	2 tablespoons baking
1½ cups milk	powder
2 eggs, beaten	1 cup chopped nuts

Combine honey, molasses, butter, milk and eggs. Sift flour, salt and baking powder. Add nuts to flour and mix in. Stir the dry ingredients into the liquid ingredients until thoroughly moistened. Pour the batter into 2 greased loaf pans and let stand 20 minutes. Bake in a 350-degree oven about an hour, until toothpick stuck into the center comes out clean. Cool before cutting, preferably on a rack of some kind to let air circulate under the bread. *Makes 2 loaves.*

BUTTERMILK NUT BREAD:
Use 1½ cups buttermilk instead of milk. Use 3 eggs. Use 1 teaspoon soda and 4 teaspoons baking powder, instead of 2 tablespoons baking powder.

CRANBERRY NUT BREAD:
Use 1 tablespoon baking powder and 1 teaspoon soda. Use orange juice instead of milk. Fold in 3 cups cranberries at the end, with 2 tablespoons grated orange or lemon rind.

WHOLE-GRAIN NUT BREAD:
Use 1 cup whole wheat flour instead of an equal amount of white. Or use 1 cup bran for 1 cup flour.

PUMPKIN NUT BREAD:

Omit milk and use 1½ cups canned or cooked pumpkin. Use 3 eggs. Add 1 teaspoon cinnamon, ½ teaspoon nutmeg, and grated rind of 1 lemon.

BANANA NUT BREAD:

Use 2 mashed bananas instead of 1 cup of the milk. Use 3 eggs. Add 1 teaspoon nutmeg.

DESSERTS

Ideally we will all get to the point where the thought of anything sweeter than a plain apple is unappealing. But most of us have been raised in a culture of sugar junkies, and that programming runs deep. Accordingly, sometimes we may want to have dessert, something more than "just a piece of fruit." So be it. Perhaps we are celebrating with friends, or perhaps we are just having a sweet tooth attack. If you must have dessert, why not make a rule that you will eat it only if you have made it at home from scratch?

That way, you can control what goes into the recipe and how much. I find that I can almost always cut the sweetener in a conventional recipe in half, and that's *after* I allow for the fact that less honey is needed than sugar. Also, if you have to stop and make your sweets from scratch every time you get the craving, it will slow you down.

Similarly, if you are having guests, agree with yourself that you'll serve only a homemade pie, or custard, or cooked apples over ice cream (delicious). And it turns out that custard made from scratch is really no more trouble than pudding out of a package.

With that in mind, recipes are offered, not because dessert is good for you, but because most of us eat it sometimes. Better ours than theirs! You'll find a couple of carob recipes for the chocoholics, instructions for fruit pies, the humble but satisfying rice pudding, and—for a quick dessert when you're pressed for time—the very easy Apples à la Mode.

CAROB CHIP OATMEAL COOKIES

A great chocolate chip substitute. Carob chips can be found in the health food store. They are made from powder derived from the carob bean, also called St. John's Bread, a Mediterranean fruit that does not share with chocolate its caffeine or fatty acid content.

2 cups flour, sifted	1 teaspoon cinnamon
1/2 teaspoon salt	2 cups rolled oats
1/2 cup butter	1/2 cup chopped walnuts
3 large eggs	1/2 cup carob chips
3 tablespoons honey	1/2 cup apple juice
1 tablespoon blackstrap molasses	(optional)
1 teaspoon vanilla extract	

Mix the flour and salt. Cream butter with eggs, honey, molasses, vanilla and cinnamon. Add to flour and mix to blend. Stir in oats, nut meats and carob chips. If mixture seems too dry, moisten with fruit juice.

Drop spoonfuls onto lightly greased cookie sheets and bake at 350 degrees for 12–15 minutes. *Makes 2–3 dozen.*

CAROB BROWNIES

Another for the reformed chocolate-eaters. The carob sweets really do satisfy that craving.

1 cup sifted flour	Pinch of salt
1 teaspoon baking powder	1/4 pound butter
	1/2 cup carob powder

⅓ cup honey   1 teaspoon vanilla
2 eggs, beaten   ½ cup broken nut meats

Mix flour, baking powder and salt. Melt butter over low heat, add carob powder and honey and blend. Beat eggs well in mixing bowl and slowly add carob mixture. Add sifted dry ingredients and mix well. Blend in vanilla and nuts. If mixture seems too dry, add a little warm water. Pour batter into a greased 8-inch pan (or pie pan) and bake at 350 degrees for half an hour, or until a toothpick inserted in center comes out clean. *Makes 12–16.*

SIMPLE VANILLA CUSTARD

Baked in individual dishes, this makes an elegant dessert for guests. And it's quick and easy.

1 quart whole milk   4 eggs
1 tablespoon honey   1 tablespoon vanilla
Pinch of salt   Nutmeg

Heat milk to boiling and scald with honey and salt; cool to warm. Beat the eggs. Slowly pour milk into eggs, stirring, and add vanilla. Beat mixture hard until frothy and pour into baking dish or custard cups. Sprinkle with grated nutmeg, and bake in a pan containing about an inch of water in a 350-degree oven for about 40 minutes, until top is golden and a knife comes out clean. Do not overcook. *Serves 6–8.*

RICE PUDDING

Simple and satisfying, a great way to use leftover rice.

1 cup cooked rice   ½ cup raisins
2 tablespoons honey   1½ cups milk

¼ teaspoon cinnamon   1 teaspoon vanilla
    Pinch of salt   Nutmeg

Combine rice, honey, raisins, milk, cinnamon, salt and vanilla
in the top of a double boiler. Place over water at a low boil,
stirring occasionally, for 15 minutes to half an hour. Garnish
with grated nutmeg.   *Serves 2–3.*

FRUIT PIES

There's hardly a more welcome dessert than homemade pie.
The hard part—and it's not that hard—is getting the hang of
the crust. If you're not a baker, read the section about baking
first.

THE CRUST:
    3 cups unbleached flour   ⅔ cup shortening
    1 teaspoon salt   1 cup ice water

THE FILLING:
    3 cups berries or other   Pinch of salt
      fruit   ¼ teaspoon cinnamon
    3 tablespoons honey   1–2 tablespoons flour
    1 tablespoon lemon
      juice

Sift the flour and the salt together. Cut in the shortening—
half Crisco and half butter makes a flaky crust—using a
pastry blender, or two knives, or a knife and a fork against
each other. When the flour resembles coarse corn meal and
the bits of shortening are the size of small peas, slowly add
just enough water to make a workable dough (one that hangs
together but isn't too sticky). You probably won't need quite
the whole cup of water, but it's handy to have it. It must be
cold. I start with tap water, add a few ice cubes, and let it sit
in the refrigerator until I need it.

Turn half the dough onto a well-floured board, dust with

flour, and roll out, using a floured rolling pin. Lay this pie shell in a pie pan (the easy way to do this without tearing the crust is gently to fold it in half and then redouble it, then unfold into pie pan). The crust should lap over the edges of the pan at least a half inch. Store this crust in the freezer while you roll out the other one. Drape it over the bottom of a pie pan and put it in the refrigerator until you're ready to assemble the pie.

Mix filling ingredients to coat fruit. Some people insist flour won't work as a thickener with acid fruit like berries and peaches, but I haven't found it a problem.

Spoon fruit into the bottom pie shell. Cover with top shell. Pinch crust edges together, fluting the edge of the pie crust by pinching it into little peaks with your fingers if you like. Cut several gashes in top crust to let steam escape, and bake at 450 degrees for 10 minutes. Reduce to 350 degrees and cook until golden brown, about half an hour. Allow to cool for at least 15 minutes before serving.   *Makes a 2-crust 9-inch pie.*

NOTE: For a good, flaky crust it is important to handle the dough as little as possible and keep the shortening cold. Also, more shortening will make a flakier and more manageable crust.

APPLES À LA MODE

A delicious, simple dessert—and much quicker than apple pie.

Peel and slice 1 small apple (Winesaps are good) per person. Put in saucepan with 2 tablespoons maple syrup per 4 apples. Sprinkle with cinnamon and grated nutmeg and cook over low heat till apples are soft (5–10 minutes), stirring once or twice. One tablespoon of rum or bourbon may go in if you have it.

Put a scoop of vanilla ice cream in each dessert dish. Top with the apples.

NOTE: Works well with other fresh fruit, of course—especially pears, peaches and berries.

YOGURT

It's really pretty easy. The trick is to use fresh yogurt with active cultures for a starter and to get the temperature right.

1 quart milk
2–3 tablespoons plain
    yogurt

Heat milk to boiling and let cool. The milk must feel warm, not hot to your wrist; 100 to 110 degrees is optimal if you have a food thermometer. Stir yogurt into milk and place in a warmed container in a warm place for 4–8 hours. *Makes 1 quart.*

NOTES: The milk must be boiled to kill unfriendly bacteria. The yogurt cultures are like yeast; the cooled milk must be warm enough to let them work but not hot enough to kill them. It helps to remember that body temperature is 98.6 degrees Fahrenheit, so 100 degrees feels just barely warm.

The container can be warmed by rinsing in hot water.

For the warm place (and warm container, all in one), the simplest thing is a Thermos. It's foolproof as far as I know. An electric yogurt maker provides you with handy storage containers, if you prefer it. I haven't had much luck with covered bowls stuck in the oven with the pilot light on, though some people do. If you want to try that way, use large, clean jars with tight-fitting lids and put them in a pan of warm water in the oven or wrap them up in towels and put in any warm place. Don't fill them right to the top; leave room for a little air in the jar or Thermos.

For a sweeter dessert yogurt, add any cooked fruit after yogurt has set.

Failed yogurt most often results from the wrong temperature—starting it too warm or too cool, or letting the yogurt sit in a draft or cool place while setting—or from unclean containers, old cultures, or adding too much culture as a starter (the yogurt smothers itself). Failed yogurt can sometimes be started all over by reheating the milk, thus killing off the yogurt cultures, and starting with new cultures.

For extra richness, non-instant dried milk may be added when heating the milk. Instant dried milk doesn't seem to work. Also, use whole milk, or skim milk that contains 2 percent or more fat, when making yogurt. The yogurt needs something to grow on.

SEVENTEEN

RECIPES FOR STAGE TWO

SOUP MEALS

Soups for Stage Two add a little variety to the basics of Stage One, but the soups from Stage One can travel right along with us. Here are two kinds of borscht for those who are looking for ways to add beets or cabbage to their diets. Miso soup is introduced. And for entertaining, there's bouillabaisse, an elegant version of the Mediterranean fisherman's soup. Don't neglect the good grain and legume soups from Stage One—barley and lentil. Add Black Bean Soup.

COLD CUCUMBER SOUP

2 small cucumbers	1 cup yogurt
½ small onion	¼ teaspoon salt
½ cup vegetable stock or water	1 teaspoon fresh mint, or ⅓ teaspoon dried
Juice of ½ lemon	Pepper

Peel cucumbers; seed them by cutting the flesh away from the core of the vegetable. Chop the cucumbers and the onion coarsely. Blend at medium speed with stock and lemon juice. Add the yogurt, salt and mint, and blend briefly. Chill for half an hour or more. Garnish with fresh ground pepper. *Serves 2.*

GARDEN VEGETABLE SOUP

Especially good in summer, when the vegetables are fresh. A meal in itself or with a green salad.

½ cup chopped onion	1 teaspoon honey
½ cup chopped celery	1 bay leaf
2 tablespoons oil	2 medium zucchini, sliced
4 large tomatoes, chopped	1 cup sliced okra (optional)
1½ cups broken green beans	1 cup corn cut off the cob
1 carrot, sliced thin	Salt and pepper
1 tablespoon chopped fresh basil	

Sauté onion and celery in the oil. Add 4 cups water, tomatoes, beans, carrot, basil, honey and bay leaf. Bring to boil, reduce heat, cover and simmer 30 minutes. Add squash, okra, if desired, and corn. Bring to boil and simmer, covered, 5 minutes, or until tender. Season with salt and pepper. *Serves 4.*

HOT UKRAINIAN BORSCHT

Many people find the earthy beet a difficult vegetable to like, but it is rich in minerals and is considered good for the blood —like nature's own Geritol. Borscht is a good way to eat your share of beets, since the sourness of the vinegar and sour milk (buttermilk or yogurt) perfectly complements the beet flavor, and takes the earthy edge off it. Serve with a hearty pumpernickel or rye bread.

3 large beets, without tops
1 large onion, chopped
1 large garlic clove, chopped
2 tablespoons butter
2 tablespoons oil
1 rib celery, chopped
1 can (1 pound) tomatoes, with liquid
¼ cup vinegar

1 teaspoon honey
1 tablespoon salt
3 large potatoes, sliced thin
½ head of cabbage, shredded (optional)
Tamari
Yogurt or buttermilk
Chopped parsley
Fresh ground black pepper

Steam beets until tender. Meanwhile, prepare other vegetables. Skin beets and slice them thin. Sauté onion and garlic in butter and oil; add celery, tomatoes, beets, vinegar, honey and salt; simmer half an hour. Meanwhile, bring 2 quarts water to a boil in a kettle and simmer potatoes until barely tender. Add beet mixture and cabbage, if desired. Bring to boil, reduce heat, and simmer half an hour. Correct seasoning, adding tamari. Garnish with 1 tablespoon yogurt (or 2 tablespoons buttermilk) per serving, chopped parsley, and fresh ground black pepper. *Makes 8–10 servings.*

NOTE: For extra iron and an authentic traditional touch, save the beet tops and add them, chopped, with or instead of the cabbage.

CABBAGE BORSCHT

Omit the beets, for a completely different and equally delicious dish. Garnish with chopped scallions instead of yogurt. This is also a traditional Eastern European meal.

JEANNE'S OKROSHKA

A cold cousin of borscht—"great as a lunch or supper on otherwise hot and hopeless days," as its author points out.

1 cup boiled or pickled beets, chopped fine (see note)	3–4 scallions, chopped fine
1 cup beet liquid	3 tablespoons fresh dill
1 cup yogurt or buttermilk	2–3 hard-boiled eggs, sliced
1 cucumber, chopped fine	

Put beets and liquid in a bowl; add yogurt or buttermilk until mixture is a bright magenta and a creamy texture. Add cucumber, scallions and dill, and chill thoroughly. Serve garnished with egg slices—and even ice cubes on really hot days—and add salt and pepper if needed. *Serves* 2.

NOTE: To cook beets, boil 3 or 4 thoroughly scrubbed beets in 2 cups water for 15–20 minutes, or until tender, then remove skins. If you use pickled beets instead, their juice adds a tangy taste.

SWEENEY'S FISH CHOWDER

A good way to use codfish, or any frozen fish fillet, if you have trouble getting good fresh fish. A New England–style chowder, good with a hearty bread or toasted cheese sandwiches.

1 medium onion, chopped	4 tablespoons butter
1 small garlic clove, minced	1 tablespoons olive oil
	2 tablespoons flour

1 quart clam juice or
    fish stock (from
    Bouillabaisse, see
    Index)
1 pound boneless fish
    fillets
3 tablespoons chopped
    parsley

1 bay leaf
    Pinch of thyme
3 medium potatoes,
    sliced
1 cup hot milk
½ cup yogurt
    Fresh ground black
    pepper

Sauté the onion and garlic in the butter and oil until translucent. Add flour, stirring constantly. Add clam juice or stock
and bring to a boil. Add fish and herbs. Bring to a boil and
simmer 15 minutes, or until fish is falling apart. Add potatoes
and simmer until tender. Add milk and stir in yogurt, removing from heat immediately. Garnish with black pepper.
Makes 4–6 servings.

BOUILLABAISSE

This elegant dish delights company and is surprisingly simple
to make. If you do not live in an area where the makings for
fresh fish stock are available or are in a hurry, use bottled
clam juice instead.

THE FISH STOCK:
    Bones and heads of
        two or three fish
    Bay leaf
3 peppercorns
    Pinch of fennel, or 2–
    3 fennel seeds

    Twist of orange peel
    Large pinch of
        saffron
    Small pinch of thyme

THE RED SAUCE:
2 large garlic cloves
3–4 medium onions,
    sliced
2 tablespoons olive oil

2 cans (28 ounces each)
    whole plum
    tomatoes
    Large pinch of basil

THE FISH:

2 dozen medium clams	½ pound scallops
1 pound medium shrimps, cleaned	3–4 pounds assorted fish fillets (see note)

Put all the ingredients for the stock in a kettle with 3–4 quarts water. Bring to boil and skim off foam. Simmer 45 minutes, or until meat falls off the bones. If you are not making stock from scratch, substitute 1 quart clam juice and 2 quarts water for the fish and water, and add the seasonings. Simmer briefly and set aside, while you make the red sauce.

For the red sauce, sauté garlic and onions in the oil until translucent. Add tomatoes, reserving the juice, and basil. Simmer until tomatoes begin to break down.

Strain the fish stock through cheesecloth to remove the bones; discard bones. Save the meat to add to the soup if you like. Combine fish stock and red sauce and simmer gently for 15 minutes to combine the flavors.

Add clams to broth and cook for 5 minutes. Then add other shellfish and fillets and cook until shrimp are pink and the fillets have disintegrated. By now the clams should be open. Traditionally, the bouillabaisse is ladled over slices of French bread in soup plates and garnished with parsley. *Serves 6–8.*

NOTE: This dish is a tradition of the French Mediterranean, where it was a staple of the fishermen, and by rights contains such delicacies as eel and octopus. This version is for more middle-of-the-road palates; it uses fillets instead of whole fish to save the guests from having to look out for bones. I think this makes a more relaxing meal. Good choices of fish for the fillets include flounder, sole, monkfish, cod, halibut, hake, snapper and haddock. Darker fish like weakfish are fine, too, but use them more sparingly. Try to get as much variety as possible by using a half pound of several different kinds.

BLACK BEAN SOUP

This rich, thick soup is a good winter meal.

2 cups black beans,
    soaked overnight
2 tablespoons oil
1 bay leaf
1 whole clove
1 tablespoon molasses
1 tablespoon vinegar
2 peppercorns

1 large onion, chopped
1 celery rib, chopped
1 carrot, chopped
Pinch of cayenne
    pepper
1 tablespoon tamari
Pinch of mace
Medium dry sherry

Rinse and drain the beans. Bring to boil with 1½ quarts water, oil, bay leaf, clove, molasses, vinegar, and peppercorns; reduce heat, and simmer 1½–2 hours. Add chopped vegetables, cayenne, tamari and mace, if desired. Add more water if needed and continue cooking until beans are tender. Purée mixture in a blender or food mill or use a rotary beater. Add 1 tablespoon sherry to each bowl just before serving. *Makes 6–8 servings.*

NOTE: The soup may also be garnished with chopped scallions, chopped hard-boiled egg, or—for a touch of elegance —thin slices of lemon and chopped parsley.

SIMPLE MISO SOUP

Seaweed
½ onion, sliced in to thin
    half-moons

2 ounces dry noodles
1 tablespoon miso
1 teaspoon tamari

Crumble a leaf or two (less than a small handful) of one or more seaweeds into 1½ cups of boiling water. Add onion; cover and let cook 20 minutes.

In another pot, bring to a boil enough water to cook the noodles and get them started. They'll be done in 5 minutes; set them aside.

In ½ cup warm water, stir miso paste till thoroughly dissolved.

Add noodles and tamari to seaweed mixture. Add miso mixture. Cover and let simmer for a minute.   *Makes 2 cups.*

COOKING GRAINS

Millet and the cracked grains take about half an hour to cook. Cook them as you would brown rice. Or cook them like pilaf by first roasting them in a skillet with a little oil (and chopped cooked onions, peppers or other vegetables, if desired), then adding water and boiling in a covered pot till liquid is absorbed and grain is tender.

Couscous is traditionally cooked by a rather complicated method involving a special steamer pot. I use millet instead. In a pinch couscous may be cooked like all the other grains.

Whole buckwheat groats and steel-cut oats take longer to cook. Cook as for rice, adding more water if needed, till tender. Or cook them in a pressure cooker.

PILAF

¼ cup chopped onion	2 tablespoons oil
½ cup green peppers or carrots (optional)	1 cup bulgur, kasha, millet or rice
Chopped parsley	

Sauté the vegetables lightly in oil. Add grain and sauté, stirring, for 2–3 minutes. Cover with water and cook, covered, till tender. Add more water if necessary.   *Makes 4 servings.*

PRESSURE-COOKED RICE

Pressure cooking is recommended because it seals the maximum nutritional value into the rice. It uses less water per cup of rice than does boiling.

| 3 cups short-grain brown rice | 4½ cups water
Pinch of salt |

Rinse the rice several times, until water is clear. Pick out any pebbles or badly broken grains.

Put water, rice and salt in cooker, and bring to pressure. Cook rice 45 minutes. Take pressure down, open, and allow rice to "air out" by gently separating it from the edge of the pot with a wooden paddle or spoon.   *Makes 6–8 servings.*

ENTRÉES

As I mentioned earlier, there's a tendency to eat too much dairy food as we stop eating meats. These entrées include some dairy dishes, but they also try to put grains and legumes more squarely in the middle of the meal, with stuffed vegetables, casseroles, and lentil dishes. In this category, too, are the soy dishes, where tofu and tempeh replace cheese (Macroroni) or meat (Tofu Shish Kebab, Meatless Moussaka). Other dishes, like Nancy Kiessling's Eggplant or tempura, make good dishes for entertaining. And don't forget basics from Stage One like lasagne and stir-fry: try using tofu in both of these, mashed up with the cheese in lasagne and cut in small cubes for the stir-fry. Or make a stir-fry with just staple vegetables and nuts for a quick and simple dinner. On evenings when there's no time to cook, Noodles Milanese get done in the time it takes to talk about it.

SHELLS AND BROCCOLI

An Italian classic, good as an entrée.

1 head broccoli	½ pound shells, cooked
3 tablespoons lemon	and drained
juice	Cayenne or hot dried
3 tablespoons olive oil	peppers (optional)
2 tablespoons butter	Parmesan cheese
3 garlic cloves, chopped	

Discard the base of the broccoli stem; cut the head and branches into bite-size pieces. Steam just until bright green, and sprinkle with lemon juice. Heat oil and butter and sauté garlic briefly. Toss with shells and broccoli, adding hot pepper if desired. Serve topped with Parmesan. *Serves 2–4.*

NOODLES MILANESE

This can be made in about 8 minutes, if you're in a hurry to make it to the movies on time. Goes well with a simple green salad.

2 cups egg noodles Butter or oil	4 fresh tomatoes, quartered
1 garlic clove, chopped	Basil
1 medium onion, chopped	2 tablespoons yogurt Salt and pepper Grated cheese

Set the noodles to cook. Heat the butter or oil and add garlic and onion. Sauté till clear and add tomatoes and basil; sauté until tomatoes disintegrate. Rinse cooked noodles under cold water; return to heat and toss briefly with the yogurt, adding salt and pepper if desired. Serve topped with tomatoes and grated cheese.   *Serves 2.*

LASAGNE FLORENTINE II

The addition of tofu to lasagne is a good way to introduce this soy product. Its texture is rather like cottage cheese; its taste is bland and faintly nutty.

Handful of spinach leaves, washed and drained	16 ounces cottage cheese (small curd) or ricotta (see note)
1 garlic clove Cooking oil	
16 ounces tofu	1 medium onion, chopped

8–10 mushrooms, cleaned
     and sliced
  2 medium zucchini,
     sliced thin
  2 teaspoons crushed
     basil leaves
8–12 lasagne noodles,
     cooked

  8 ounces mozzarella,
     grated
  2 eggs
  4 ounces plain yogurt
    Parmesan cheese

Sauté the spinach and garlic together in a small amount of oil. Shred fine with a knife and fork, or in a blender. Mash the tofu and the cottage cheese together and mix in the spinach. Sauté the onion, mushrooms, zucchini, and basil in a little oil (you can re-use the spinach pan). Grease a 9-by-12 baking dish and line the bottom with a layer of noodles. Spread half the tofu mixture on the noodles, and top with all of the zucchini mixture. Top this with half the mozzarella and another layer of noodles. Spread on the rest of the tofu mixture and top with the rest of the mozzarella.

Beat the eggs and yogurt together and pour over the lasagne. Sprinkle with Parmesan and bake in a 350-degree oven until top is nicely browned. *About 6 servings.*

NOTES: Cottage cheese can be lower in fat than ricotta—read the label. Ricotta provides a better texture.

If half-and-half tofu and cheese is too much at first, adjust the proportions.

RATATOUILLE-TOFU LASAGNE

8–10 whole wheat lasagne
     noodles, cooked
  2 cups leftover
     ratatouille
1½ cups ricotta

1½ cups tofu
  1 cup grated hard
     cheese
  2 eggs
½ cup yogurt

Line the bottom of a greased 9-by-9 baking pan with lasagne noodles. Cover with the ratatouille.

Mash together the ricotta and tofu. Spread one half of the mixture over the ratatouille and sprinkle on half of the hard cheese. Add a second layer of noodles. Top with the remaining tofu and ricotta. Beat the eggs and yogurt together and pour over the last layer. Top with remaining hard cheese and bake 20–30 minutes in a 350-degree oven till nicely browned. *Makes 4 servings.*

PERFECT PESTO

2 ounces fresh locatelli or Parmesan
¼–½ cup olive oil
1 or 2 whole garlic cloves, peeled
2 cups fresh or frozen basil leaves, or ½ cup dried crushed leaves

1 egg, raw or boiled 1 minute
¼ cup walnuts, pecans or other nuts
1–2 tablespoons lemon juice
½ teaspoon tamari

Break the cheese into chunks and blend or process it with the oil and the garlic on a medium setting. Add the basil and the egg, and blend coarsely. Add the walnuts and blend into a paste. Remove from blender or processor and stir in lemon juice to taste. Add tamari to taste. *Makes 2 cups; 4 servings.*

NOTES: It took me a long time and many disappointing batches to arrive at this recipe. In the first batches, I followed standard recipes, which called for far more oil and cheese, and I got a greasy pesto that made the spaghetti taste mostly of oil. Also, the basil had the sharp, bruised taste of chopped leaves. And the standard pine nuts were too expensive. By adding the egg, I seem to have compensated with extra liquid for a good half to two-thirds of the oil. Although I am a garlic lover, I use only one large clove, not to overpower the basil. By blending the oil, cheese and garlic first and then adding the egg with the basil, I seemed to avoid bruising the basil leaves (frankly, I've had the best results with frozen leaves, added while still unthawed).

I use walnuts because they're my favorites; pecan or almonds would do if you prefer them. I think it's silly to insist on the expensive pignoli—the others provide good texture and flavor and are less oily, too. For added nuttiness, crumble in half a handful after blending.

The pesto can be tossed with hot, lightly buttered pasta, or used as a dip or spread.

MONKFISH NEWBURG

The monkfish has been popularized in these inflationary days as "poor-man's lobster," hence the inspiration for this dish. Serve over rice or hot buttered toast, with a salad of lettuce and endive.

1 pound monkfish, filleted	¼ cup dry sherry
	½ teaspoon paprika
5 tablespoons butter	3 egg yolks
Juice of ½ lemon	½ cup yogurt

Pan-poach the monkfish in 2 tablespoons of the butter for 10 minutes; add the lemon juice. In a double boiler, melt the remaining 3 tablespoons butter. Cut up the monkfish and add it to the double boiler, with the sherry and paprika. Cook gently about 2 minutes. Beat egg yolks and yogurt together and stir into the mixture, cooking to thicken. Do not allow to boil. If mixture needs more liquid, heat the pan juices from the monkfish until warm, not boiling, and stir in. Serve at once. *Makes 4 servings.*

NOTE: Mushrooms make a nice addition. If you want to add them, clean and slice 10 or 12, cook them with the monkfish, and add them at the same time.

MACROTUNA CASSEROLE

1 cup Veggie-Bow or other macaroni	2 tablespoons flour
1 6-ounce can tuna, drained	1 cup skim milk
2 ounces tofu, crumbled	2 ounces mild Cheddar cheese, grated
2 tablespoons butter	2–4 ounces cottage cheese
	Bread crumbs
	Parmesan cheese

Put the macaroni on to boil. Put the tuna in a casserole dish and mix in the tofu.

Melt butter in a saucepan, stir in flour and, still stirring, slowly add milk, thickening the mixture over a low flame. Still stirring, add the Cheddar and cottage cheese to form a cheese sauce. Remove from heat.

Drain the cooked macaroni and rinse. Mix into the tuna mixture and cover with the cheese sauce. Top with bread crumbs and Parmesan, if desired. Bake in a 375-degree oven until browned, about 15 minutes. *Makes 4 servings.*

MACRORONI

A lighter dish than the traditional macaroni and cheese because of the tofu.

2 cups cooked whole wheat macaroni	1 carrot, chopped
½ pound tofu	1 small onion, chopped
½ cup grated Cheddar	Bread crumbs
1 rib celery, chopped	1 egg
	1 cup milk

Mix the macaroni, tofu, cheese and vegetables in a greased baking dish. Sprinkle with bread crumbs. Beat egg and milk together and pour over the macaroni mixture. Bake at 350 degrees for half an hour. *Makes 4 servings.*

VEGETABLE QUICHE WITH TOFU

A nice light dinner with a green salad.

2–3 tablespoons butter	½ cup mashed tofu
1 garlic clove, chopped	1 handful of spinach leaves
1 small onion, chopped	Pinch of basil
1 spear of broccoli, chopped	8 large eggs
1 zucchini, chopped	2 unbaked 9-inch pie shells
3–4 mushrooms, sliced	
1 cup grated cheese	

Melt 1 tablespoon of the butter in a skillet; sauté garlic and onion. Add broccoli, sauté lightly, and add the squash and mushrooms. Sauté lightly, adding more butter if needed. Remove from pan. Mix the grated cheese and the tofu; toss with the vegetables. Sauté the spinach and basil in the skillet, adding more butter if needed. Chop it fine. (You can chop it right in the pan, using a knife and fork in opposition.) Remove from heat and add to vegetable mixture.

Beat the eggs and add the cooled vegetables. Pour into pie shells, leaving about three-quarter inch room to rise in each pan. Bake at 375 degrees for 30 minutes, or until nicely browned. *Serves 4–6.*

ZUCCHINI-FETA CASSEROLE

A quiche-like dish that goes well as a main dish or appetizer.

- 3 small zucchini, grated
- 3 eggs
- 6 scallions, chopped
- ½ cup chopped fresh mint and/or dill weed
- ½ cup chopped parsley
- ½ cup grated feta cheese
- ½ cup grated mild cheese
- ½ cup flour
- Pinch of salt
- Pinch of cayenne pepper
- 4 tablespoons butter

Mix zucchini, eggs, scallions, mint, dill, parsley and cheeses. Add flour slowly, mixing well. Season with salt and cayenne pepper. Grease a 9-inch baking pan with 1 tablespoon of the butter. Pour in zucchini mixture. Dot with remaining butter. Bake 45 minutes at 350 degrees, until well browned. Cut into squares. Serve hot or cold. *Makes 6–8 servings.*

CHEESE AND LENTIL LOAF

A great entrée and good for sandwiches next day. Rice and cooked greens make good side dishes.

- 2 cups cooked lentils, drained
- ½ pound cheese, grated
- 1 small onion, chopped
- 1 tablespoon tamari
- ¼ teaspoon fresh ground black pepper
- ¼ teaspoon thyme
- 1 cup bread crumbs
- 1 egg, beaten
- 1 tablespoon soft butter or oil

Mash lentils, cheese and onion together. Add remaining ingredients and mix thoroughly.

Bake in greased loaf pan 45 minutes at 350 degrees. *Makes 5–6 servings.*

NOTE: For a more meatloaf-like effect, top the loaf with a brushing of Dijon mustard or a half cup of Basic Marinara Sauce (see Index), spread evenly.

LENTIL BURGERS

2 cups cooked lentils	1 egg, beaten
⅓ cup finely diced sautéed nuts and vegetables	2 teaspoons soy sauce Oatmeal or rolled oats 1 tablespoon oil

THE VEGETABLES:
Chop very fine small amounts of your favorite vegetables—carrots, celery, onions and mushrooms are good; so are peppers, squash and eggplant—and sauté in a little oil with finely chopped nuts.

Mash together the lentils and the cooked vegetables. Stir in the egg and the soy sauce. Add enough uncooked oatmeal or rolled oats so that the mixture will stick together. Shape into patties, separating patties in layers with wax paper, and chill on a plate in the refrigerator half an hour. Sauté in oil on both sides until crisp. *Makes 4 patties.*

CHEESEBURGERS:
After turning the lentil burgers, top with a slice of cheese. Serve the burgers in pita pockets with lettuce, sliced tomato and onion.

LENTIL LOAF:
Prepare Lentil Burger mixture. Bake in a greased loaf pan at 350 degrees for half an hour. For a crustier loaf, brush top with an egg, beaten with 1 teaspoon tamari.

TEMPEH LOAF

A delicious non-meat loaf.

1 pound tempeh Rolled oats as needed	1 slice daikon radish, chopped
1 egg	1 small shiitake
2 tablespoons tamari	mushroom, soaked
1 tablespoon ginger juice	and chopped
1 carrot, grated	¼ green pepper, chopped
1 onion, chopped fine	1 tablespoon prepared
1 rib celery, chopped	mustard

THE GLAZE:

1 tablespoon oil	1 tablespoon prepared
2 tablespoons tamari	mustard

Mash loaf ingredients together, adding as much rolled oats as needed to make mixture stick together. Shape it into a loaf and bake in a greased pie tin at 350 degrees for 45 minutes. Combine glaze ingredients and brush top of loaf occasionally with glaze. Allow to cool 5–10 minutes before slicing. Serve with Mushroom Gravy (recipe follows).   *Serves 4.*

MUSHROOM GRAVY

1 large shiitake mushroom	2 teaspoons oil
½ onion, sliced	1 tablespoon kudzu or
1 small carrot, chopped	arrowroot powder,
2 tablespoons tamari	dissolved in cold
1 cup sliced fresh mushrooms	water

Simmer the shiitake, sliced onion, carrot and tamari in 3 cups water for 10 minutes or more. Remove shiitake, slice fine (discarding stem), and replace. Sauté fresh mushrooms in oil and add to the stock. Add dissolved thickener and simmer, stirring constantly, until liquid is clear and slightly thickened.

NOTE: Serve over any non-meat loaf.

NANCY KIESSLING'S EGGPLANT

An excellent main dish. Serve with rice and a salad if desired.

4 ½-inch slices eggplant	1 hard-boiled egg,
4 tablespoons butter	chopped
½ green pepper, cut into	Parsley
quarters	
1 large tomato, sliced	
2 tablespoons Deluxe	
Bread Crumbs (see	
Index)	

Sauté the eggplant in 2 tablespoons of the butter in a large saucepan. Reserve. Add remaining butter to pan; sauté the pepper. When nearly done, add the tomatoes and grill lightly, so as not to break them. Top each slice of eggplant with a slice of tomato and a slice of pepper. Set in a baking dish.

Put the bread crumbs into the saucepan in which the vegetables were cooked and heat to absorb any remaining juices or butter. Sprinkle over each stack of vegetables and grill briefly under the broiler. Garnish with hard-cooked egg, and parsley, if desired. *Makes 4 servings.*

STUFFED PEPPERS

A hearty entrée.

6 green peppers	1 tablespoon basil
1 small onion, chopped	1 teaspoon curry powder
2 medium tomatoes	1 teaspoon gomasio
½ cup chopped nuts	2 tablespoons parsley
2 tablespoons oil	Tamari to taste
1 cup chopped mushrooms	A handful of small cubes of mild cheese
1 tablespoon butter	
1½ cup cooked rice or other grain	6 small slices sharp Cheddar or Swiss cheese
1 teaspoon dried dill weed	
1 tablespoon oregano	

Steam whole peppers till almost tender (the color will start to fade). Cut off tops and remove seed core. Sauté onion, tomatoes and nuts in oil. Sauté mushrooms in butter. Mix vegetables, rice, seasonings and cheese cubes. Stuff peppers and top with slices of cheese. Bake 20–25 minutes at 350 degrees. *Serves 4–6.*

STUFFED WINTER SQUASH

An entrée or a side dish.

2 squashes, split and cleaned	6 mushrooms, chopped
Butter	1 small carrot, cut into matchsticks
Nutmeg	Tamari
Cinnamon	¼ cup nut meats, chopped
1 small onion, chopped	1 cup cooked rice
½ cup shredded cabbage	

Bake the squash, split side down, in a greased pan for about
20 minutes at 350 degrees. Turn over, put a pat of butter in
the hollow of each half and sprinkle with nutmeg and cinnamon. Return to oven, face up.

Sauté the vegetables, adding tamari and nuts after about a
minute or two. Toss with rice.

Remove squashes from oven and gently cut the squash
meat away from the shell. Chop the squash meat coarsely and
combine it with vegetable-rice mixture. Return to squash
shells and serve.   *Makes 4 servings.*

ALMOND CABBAGE ROLLS

Serve these hearty bundles of protein as an entrée with salad
or baked squash on the side.

8 large cabbage leaves	2 tablespoons Parmesan
2 medium onions,	cheese
chopped	½ cup chopped almonds
½ green pepper,	Tomato-Dill Sauce
chopped	(recipe follows)
3 tablespoons oil	Sour cream or yogurt
3 cups cooked brown	
rice	
1 cup Cheddar or	
Monterey Jack	
cheese	

Blanch whole cabbage leaves for several minutes, until just
flexible. Rinse in cold water, drain, and cut out thick rib
section so leaves will lie flat.

Sauté onion and green pepper in 1 tablespoon of the oil to
brown; add rice and stir in. Remove from heat and toss with
cheeses and almonds. Divide rice mixture among cabbage
leaves and roll up, securing with toothpicks.

Heat 2 tablespoons oil and brown cabbage rolls lightly,

carefully turning once. Pour sauce over the rolls and simmer, covered, for 25 minutes. When rolls are ready to serve, top each with a teaspoon of sour cream or yogurt. Garnish with chopped almonds. *Makes 8 servings.*

TOMATO-DILL SAUCE

3 cups Basic Marinara Sauce (see Index)	1 tablespoon dill Pinch of black pepper
3 tablespoons lemon juice	

Mix all ingredients together.

WILD RICE CASSEROLE

Wild rice—not a rice at all, but the seed of a grass native to the northern wetlands of the United States—is expensive, but its texture is a treat, and like other seeds, it is rich in protein. The mixture of brown rice and wild rice cuts the expense. Serve this casserole as a main dish.

⅓ cup wild rice	1 small zucchini, cut into matchsticks
⅓ cup brown rice	
½ teaspoon salt	½ cup broccoli florets
1 carrot, cut into matchsticks	10–12 mushrooms, sliced
1 onion, chopped	1 cup grated mild cheese
1 rib celery, chopped	¼ cup sliced almonds

Rinse the rices and cook them together with salt in 2 cups water. Meanwhile, steam the vegetables briefly, 2–5 minutes. Toss rices and vegetables and turn them into a shallow baking dish. Top with cheese and nuts and cook under broiler until cheese melts. *Serves 4–6.*

BEAN AND SQUASH CHOWDER

A nice rich dish for a winter supper.

2 cups navy beans, soaked overnight	1 tablespoon tamari
1 large onion, chopped	½ teaspoon oregano
2 tablespoons paprika	1 acorn squash, peeled, seeded and chopped
3 tablespoons olive oil	½ cup corn kernels
4 medium fresh or canned tomatoes	Tabasco sauce (optional)

Rinse and drain beans. Cook in water to cover for 1½ hours. Meanwhile, sauté onion and paprika together in olive oil, 5–7 minutes. Add tomatoes, tamari and oregano and cook until well blended. Add tomato sauce and squash to the beans and cook until squash begins to disintegrate and thicken the sauce. Add corn and cook 5 minutes. Serve in soup plates and garnish with Tabasco, if desired.   *Makes 4–6 servings.*

BEANS WITH RICE

1 cup kidney or black beans	Tamari
1 medium onion, sliced	1 tablespoon molasses
2 garlic cloves, chopped	Other herbs (optional)
1 bay leaf	1 cup rice, rinsed and drained

Soak beans overnight; discard water and rinse. Add beans to 1 quart boiling water with onion, garlic and bay leaf and boil 1 hour. Add tamari and molasses and other herbs, if desired. Stir, cook 5 minutes, and add rice; stir it in, bring to a boil, and cook over low heat until all liquid is absorbed and rice is tender. *Serves 4.*

NOTES: When this dish is made Cuban-style, saffron is often one of the extra seasonings, and black beans are used to make an elegant contrast with the yellow rice. You can also, of course, use any other beans you like.

You may find "real" beans something of a shock, if you are used to canned—the canned have sugar in them, and the beans made from scratch will seem earthier and of course not as sweet. That's where the molasses comes in, and the tamari also adds flavor.

If you find intestinal gas a problem with beans, follow the cooking method in Stage Three, using seaweed (see Index for Basic Beans). It really helps!

HOPPIN' JOHN

An adaptation of Fawn Vrazo's rendering of this traditional Southern dish, which originated in the West Indies, is a great way to use black-eyed peas. In the South, the black-eyed pea was ubiquitous as a poor man's dish, and to this day is considered to bring good luck if eaten on New Year's Day. Good as a main or side dish.

8 ounces dried black-eyed peas, soaked overnight
1 cup rice soaked in cold water 30 minutes and drained
1 teaspoon salt
1 medium onion, chopped
1 tablespoon oil
1 can (1 pound) tomatoes, with liquid
¼ teaspoon cayenne pepper
½ teaspoon black pepper
1 teaspoon tamari

Drain and rinse the peas and bring to boil with 6 cups water
in a large pan. Reduce heat and simmer, covered, for 1½
hours. Add the rice and salt and continue cooking. Meanwhile, sauté the onion in oil and add the tomatoes, cayenne,
black pepper and tamari. Pour mixture into the pot with rice
and peas and stir to mix. Cook another 15–20 minutes, or
until rice and peas are tender.   *Makes 4–6 servings.*

MEATLESS CHILI

A good way to practice cooking your beans, grain and
tempeh. Serve with brown rice or corn bread.

THE BEANS:

2 cups kidney beans	1 bay leaf
1 cup aduki beans	2 teaspoons sea salt

THE SAUCE:

2 onions, chopped	Basic Chili Powder
2 garlic cloves, chopped	(recipe follows)
1 small green pepper, chopped	1 can (1 pound) tomatoes, drained (reserve juice)
Oil	
½ pound tempeh, marinated in ½ cup tamari and ½ cup water for ½ hour	¼ cup vinegar and/or wine

Rinse the beans separately and soak them separately overnight. Discard soaking water and rinse. Bring two quarts
fresh water to a boil. Then cook kidney beans for an hour.
Add aduki beans and bay leaf and cook half an hour. Add salt
and cook another half hour or until tender.

Sauté onion, garlic and green pepper in the oil. Add
tempeh and sauté until lightly browned. Stir in chili powder.
Add tomatoes and simmer half an hour or more, using the
juice to dilute if the mixture seems dry. Combine the sauce

and the beans, add vinegar or wine, and simmer 10 minutes. *Makes 6–8 servings.*

NOTES: Chili is certainly a personal taste. Great disputes rage at annual cookoffs as to whether real chili has tomatoes in it. Some like it hot. Some don't. Some eat it in bowls like soup, others eat it over rice. Only you can decide how hot (cayenne) and acid (tomatoes, vinegar) to make it.

Other good additions are fresh hot (jalapeño) peppers (instead of the cayenne); a teaspoon of filé powder or ground sassafras root; a teaspoon or more of blackstrap molasses.

BASIC CHILI POWDER

1–2 tablespoons ground cumin	1 teaspoon cardamom
1 teaspoon coriander	½ teaspoon cayenne pepper

Blend ingredients until well combined.

MEATLESS MOUSSAKA

8 ounces tempeh	Small handful of broken nut meats
¾ cup Marinade (recipe follows)	1 can (1 pound) whole plum tomatoes, drained (reserve liquid)
1 medium eggplant Butter or olive oil	
1 medium onion, chopped	Honey or molasses (optional)
1 large garlic clove, chopped	1 cup bread crumbs
8–10 large mushrooms, sliced	1 beaten egg
½ teaspoon black pepper	8 ounces ricotta
½ cup fresh chopped parsley	4 ounces yogurt
1 teaspoon cinnamon	4 ounces grated cheese
	Nutmeg

Marinate the tempeh for several hours.

Prepare the eggplant by slicing into thin rounds and quickly sautéing all of it until brown in small amounts of butter or oil. Remove from pan and set aside.

Sauté the onion and garlic in the same pan in 2 tablespoons butter or oil. Add the mushrooms and sauté.

Drain the tempeh and crumble it into the pan, so that it has the consistency of ground beef. Sauté with the onions and mushrooms over high heat for several minutes. Add pepper, parsley, cinnamon and nut meats and stir in.

Add the tomatoes and break them up. Sauté, adding tomato liquid and some of the marinade, to taste. If necessary, sweeten with honey or molasses slightly to balance the tomatoes. Simmer, adding more liquid if necessary, until the tomatoes are a sauce, 15–30 minutes.

Put a fine layer of bread crumbs in the bottom of a greased 9-by-9 pan. Add a layer of eggplant, then a layer of the tempeh mixture. Repeat until all is used.

Beat the egg, ricotta and yogurt together. Pour over the moussaka. Top with grated cheese. Sprinkle with grated nutmeg if desired. Bake at 375 degrees half an hour or until golden brown. *Makes 4–6 servings.*

NOTES: Like many casseroles, moussaka improves with sitting; if possible, make it a day in advance and refrigerate.

The eggplant, a real glutton for oil, will soak up all you give it and demand more. Put in your butter or oil a little at a time and stir through the eggplant on as high a heat as you can use without burning. The slices will even absorb fat from each other if they are in contact, so what at first looks like a hopeless amount of naked vegetable does soon become oily, browned and limp.

This dish will never be a real moussaka substitute for the dedicated lamb lover. But it does offer the good flavors of tomato, onion, mushroom and eggplant and the meaty texture of the tempeh against the fluffy cheese crust.

MARINADE

¾ cup white wine (or ½
　　cup white wine and
　　¼ cup sherry)
1 crushed garlic clove

½ teaspoon grated
　　ginger
1 teaspoon tamari

Blend all ingredients in a bowl.

SKEWERED TOFU WITH PEANUT SAUCE

An excellent dish for a cookout. Marinate in advance and take it along to barbecues where you know meat will be served. Best cooked over charcoal, though the tofu can also be cooked under a broiler. The skewers that work best are the very thin bamboo ones, which can be purchased at Oriental groceries or at some gourmet food stores. For a complete meal, serve with Hoppin' John (see Index) and a salad of lettuce and mustard greens.

1 pound tofu, cut
　　lengthwise into
　　strips
　Juice of 1 lemon
3 tablespoons soy sauce
　1-inch piece of ginger,
　　grated

1 tablespoon oil
1 garlic clove, minced
　Peanut Sauce (recipe
　　follows)

Marinate the tofu in the lemon juice, soy sauce, ginger, oil and garlic for half an hour to an hour, turning once or twice.

Meanwhile, prepare Peanut Sauce and start the charcoal. When tofu is ready, cook over charcoal (or under broiler), basting with marinade several times, for about 10 minutes. Serve with Peanut Sauce. *Serves 3–4.*

PEANUT SAUCE

This is adapted from a recipe contributed by John Vrazo, who serves it with barbecued pork. The original recipe comes from *This Is the Way We Cook (Asina Nos Ta Cushina)*, featuring recipes from the Netherlands Antilles.

3 large onions	1 tablespoon molasses
4 tablespoons oil	1 tablespoon honey
1 teaspoon Tabasco sauce	Juice of 2 limes
1 cup peanuts	2 tablespoons roasted sesame seeds
2 garlic cloves	Milk (optional)
3 tablespoons soy sauce	

Slice 2 of the onions and sauté in the oil. Mince the remaining onion, sprinkle with the Tabasco sauce, and set aside. In a blender or food mill, thoroughly mix all of the ingredients except the Tabasco–raw onion mixture. Pour the sauce from the blender into a saucepan and boil over low heat. The sauce should be textured and rather thick, but if it appears too thick, add water, a little at a time, stirring. If oil appears on the surface, add a few tablespoons of milk. Remove from heat and stir in the Tabasco–raw onion mixture. Serve over grilled tofu or on the side.

TOFU SHISH KEBAB

Good for picnics.

1 pound tofu, cubed and marinated	2 peppers, cut into pieces
Marinade (recipe follows)	2 onions, quartered
3 tomatoes, quartered	12 mushroom caps

Marinate the tofu cubes in marinade for at least an hour.
Then thread on skewers with the vegetables and broil or cook
over charcoal. Enough for 6–8 skewers.

MARINADE

½ cup lemon juice	1 tablespoon tamari
½ teaspoon fresh grated ginger	1 tablespoon oil

Mix and pour over the tofu cubes.

SPANAKOPITA

A variant of the Greek original. Serve with brown rice and
salad.

1 pound spinach or other dark greens	3 eggs
1 garlic clove, chopped	1 cup grated mild cheese
Oil	Basic Biscuits recipe, doubled (see Index)
1 tablespoon tamari	
1 pound tofu, crumbled	

Wash and drain spinach and sauté briefly with garlic in oil.
Stir in tamari, tofu, eggs and cheese. Make biscuit dough and
split in half.

Roll out bottom crust very thin on floured board or counter
top. Crust should be large enough for a pizza pan, cookie
sheet or large baking pan.

Fold dough gently in quarters to remove from board. Unfold into pan. Roll out top crust. Spread spinach mixture onto
bottom crust, leaving a 1-inch margin. Cover with top crust
and pinch edges of crusts together. Gash upper crust in several places to release steam. Brush with melted butter if
desired. Bake at 400 degrees for 40 minutes, or until brown.

Cut in squares or wedges. *Makes a main course for 6, or hors d'oeuvres for many.*

NOTE: If desired, split dough into 6–8 portions, roll out each and fill, folding over to make turnovers.

DEEP-FRIED DISHES

Deep-frying is a useful technique for a variety of festive finger foods, from hors d'oeuvres (egg rolls, falafel) to entrées (tempura).

It helps to have a deep-frying thermometer, but if you don't, a good test of the heat of the fat is to drop a cube of bread into the fryer (which can be any heavy pot deep enough to hold several inches of oil comfortably without spattering you or the kitchen). If the bread rises to the surface and crisps to a golden brown within a minute, the oil is hot enough. If the oil starts to smoke, it is too hot; try to avoid this.

When the fat is ready, drop in a few of the items you are frying—not too many at a time or you'll crowd the fryer and cause the fat temperature to drop. When the food rises to the surface and turns golden, remove with a slotted spoon or an Oriental skimmer. (If you have a conventional deep fryer, it has a basket that makes retrieving the fried food quite convenient, but this is not essential.) Drain the food on paper toweling on top of a brown paper bag, and serve at once.

Good quality safflower oil is a good, light oil for deep frying, though sesame is often used in Oriental cooking. You may want to try a mixture—say 75 percent safflower and 25 percent light-weight sesame. Chinese recipes often call for peanut oil, which has a delightful flavor but is less easily digested.

After cooking, cool the oil and pour through a sieve; store it in the refrigerator, and you may use it several times.

EGG ROLLS

THE FILLING:

1 cup shredded cabbage	½ cup broken nut meats,
1 small onion, finely chopped	or ½ cup finely chopped shrimp
½ cup diced peppers, carrots and mushrooms	1 tablespoon tamari
	1 cup cooked grain

THE WRAPPERS:

2 cups flour	1 tablespoon oil
3 cups water	2 eggs

Prepare the filling by lightly sautéing the vegetables and nut meats or shrimp in oil. Add the tamari at the end of the sautéing, which should take 2–3 minutes. Add to grain and mix in.

Prepare the batter for the wrappers as you would pancake batter. The wrapper will actually be a crêpe cooked on one side only, so the batter should be thin enough to pour easily; adjust water to achieve desired consistency.

Pour enough batter into a greased pan (a small frying pan is ideal) barely to cover the pan, tipping pan to spread the batter evenly. Let it cook briefly, then tip it onto a plate, cooked side up, or lift it out quickly with your fingers and lay it cooked side up. Repeat, stacking the wrappers.

Now fill each wrapper with the filling, folding them securely like little envelopes, which you seal with a paste made of flour and water (just mix up a couple of tablespoons of each in a cup). Use just a little paste for each wrapper. The *uncooked* side of the wrapper is now on the outside.

Deep fry the egg rolls, drain and serve. If you prefer a less greasy egg roll, brush with oil *or* water and bake in a 350-degree oven on a greased cookie sheet until nicely browned —about 10 minutes. *Makes 10–12.*

NOTE: If you are baking the egg rolls, you may also try brushing them with egg yolk beaten with 2 tablespoons water.

For the filling, varying ingredients may be used—whatever combination of vegetables, grain and other protein (including beans or seeds) you fancy.

Commercially made egg-roll wrappers by Nasoya are now available in grocery stores.

FALAFEL

Falafel is a traditional Middle Eastern snack and is an ideal hors d'oeuvre at parties. A few falafels—or one falafel patty, if you make a large one—will make an ideal filling for a pita-bread sandwich with fresh greens or other raw vegetables. If you like a spicier falafel, add minced garlic and a dash of cayenne pepper.

¾ cup cooked chick-peas
¼ cup tahini (sesame paste)
¼ cup finely chopped onion (and/or carrots, celery, parsley)

Flour
Oil for cooking

Mash chick-peas, tahini and onion together and form into 1-inch balls. Dredge these in flour and deep fry at 350 degrees (or in oil that is hot enough to lightly brown a test cube of bread). *Makes 12 or more.*

NOTE: If you don't want to deep fry them, the mixture can be pressed into patties instead and sautéed.

BEER-BATTER TEMPURA

Inspired by a picnic at the Conlows' home, where the tempura started out as an appetizer and proved so popular that no one had room for the hamburgers. The batter should be prepared a few hours in advance and left to stand and rest, refrigerated. This allows a mild fermentation (increased by the beer), which improves the texture of the batter. The egg yolks help the batter resist the fat during deep-frying. Egg whites, if desired, may be added, stiffly beaten, just before cooking. This dish, one of the "fast foods" of the Orient, may be the trendy party food of the future. Does anybody remember fondue?

THE BATTER:

1 cup unbleached flour	2 egg yolks, beaten
1 teaspoon salt	¾ cup flat beer
Pinch of pepper	2 egg whites (optional)
1 tablespoon oil	

Combine flour, salt, pepper, oil and egg yolks. Add beer, stirring constantly. Batter should be just shy of runny. Refrigerate 3–12 hours. Add egg whites, beaten stiff, just before cooking, if desired.

THE VEGETABLES:

Up to 2 cups raw vegetables cut in bite-size pieces. Carrot and squash slices, broccoli florets, onion rings, strips of bell pepper and mushrooms are favorites.

The vegetables should be free of moisture. Pat dry if necessary. Heat the frying oil, at least several inches deep, in a kettle that is at least twice as deep as the oil. (The diameter of the pot is not important, although it governs how many pieces you fry at once, but the pot should be sturdy and deep enough.)

When the oil is about 350 degrees (a small cube of bread

will be golden brown after one minute), reduce heat to medium-high, dip vegetables in batter, and commence frying.

Drain the pieces on paper towels if you can keep your
fellow diners at bay. Recommended sauces:

SOY DIPPING SAUCE

½ cup tamari
    grated or dry ginger

2 tablespoons lemon
    juice

Mix all ingredients in a bowl.

MUSTARD SAUCE

4 tablespoons Dijon or
    hot Chinese
    mustard

2 tablespoons rice
    vinegar
1 garlic clove, mashed

Mix all ingredients in a bowl.

SWEET SAUCE

¼ cup any fruit compote
    or preserve
    (chutney is good
    too)

2 tablespoons fruit juice
2 tablespoons water
    Dash of cinnamon
    (optional)

Mix all ingredients in a bowl.

SIDE DISHES AND SALADS

A couple of additional ideas for salads and other vegetable dishes—Cooked Greens is just a reminder to eat a dark green vegetable every day; Greek Salad can be a meal in itself. Marinated Vegetables are good for a buffet dinner or a summer meal.

BEAN SALAD

A variant of the traditional three-bean salad, with a touch of the cumin beloved of people who live in hot climates. A great side dish for any casserole. Good for picnics, too.

- 1 cup broken and cooked green beans
- 1 cup cooked or canned kidney beans
- 1 cup cooked or canned chick-peas
- 3 tablespoons olive oil
- 3 tablespoons wine or rice vinegar

- Pinch of salt and pepper
- 1 tablespoon chopped parsley
- ¼ teaspoon cumin
- 1 small onion, chopped fine

Toss all the ingredients together and chill at least half an hour. *Makes 6 or more servings.*

NOTE: The green beans must be fresh, not canned, to make the salad what it ought to be. Steam them until crisp-tender. The dish is improved by tossing it together while the green beans are still warm.

FRENCH POTATO SALAD

A wonderful version of this picnic favorite. Serve as a side dish with your Lentil Burgers (see Index) or grilled fish.

6 small potatoes, boiled and sliced thin
1 small onion, chopped fine
1 garlic clove, mashed
⅓ cup olive oil
3 tablespoons wine or rice vinegar
1 teaspoon dried tarragon
Salt and fresh ground black pepper
1 hard-boiled egg (optional)

Slice the potatoes when they are as hot as you can stand them. While still warm, toss potatoes with onion, garlic, oil, vinegar and tarragon. Season sparingly with salt and garnish with black pepper and, if desired, sliced egg. Serve chilled. *Makes 6 servings.*

TABBOULEH SALAD WITH MILLET

2 tomatoes
1 cup cooked millet, cooled
¼ cup minced onions
1 cup finely chopped parsley
½ cup chopped mint leaves
¼ cup lemon juice
¼ cup oil
2 teaspoons gomasio
Lettuce

Cut the tomatoes in half, crosswise. Gently squeeze out seeds. Chop tomatoes fine and set aside to drain.

Toss the millet with the other ingredients except the lettuce. Just before serving, drain excess juice from tomatoes

and add them to the salad. Toss gently and taste. Adjust
seasoning if necessary. Serve on a bed of lettuce.   *Serves 2.*

NOTE: Traditionally, this dish is made with bulgur wheat. It
is good with any of the cracked grains.

To use bulgur, simply soak ½ cup bulgur for 45 minutes.
Drain it through cheesecloth or a clean dish towel, squeezing
to remove excess liquid.

GREEK SALAD

1 small head lettuce, washed and drained	Fresh parsley, chopped
2 tomatoes	Fresh mint (optional)
1 small cucumber, sliced	½ pound feta cheese
Small jar hot green peppers	½ cup olive oil
Small jar Greek olives	¼ cup vinegar
	Salt and pepper

Tear lettuce and combine with vegetables and herbs in a
large bowl. Crumble feta cheese over salad and toss with oil.
Add vinegar, toss, taste, and add salt and pepper as desired.
Makes 4–6 servings.

EGG AND TOFU SALAD

3 hard-boiled eggs	Pinch of black pepper
½-inch slice tofu, mashed	Salt
1 tablespoon lemon juice	1 celery rib, chopped fine
1 teaspoon oil, or 2 teaspoons mayonnaise	¼ cup chopped nuts

Mix ingredients, mashing egg and tofu together first. Garnish with lettuce and/or alfalfa sprouts and spread on sandwiches or serve plain. *Makes 4 servings.*

GUACAMOLE

1 ripe avocado	Pinch of cayenne
2 tablespoons lemon juice	1 teaspoon cumin
1 garlic clove, mashed	Mayonnaise

Mash or blend all ingredients except mayonnaise. Put avocado mixture in a bowl and spread with a thin layer of mayonnaise (this prevents avocado from discoloring). Chill until just before serving, then stir in mayonnaise. Serve as an hors d'oeuvre or spread on sandwiches and add lettuce, tomato and/or sprouts. Good in Taco Salad (see Index). *Makes sandwiches for 2.*

MACARONI SALAD

A good lunch, with or without a scoop of cottage cheese on the side.

2 cups cooked macaroni	1 cucumber, sliced
½ cup cubed mild cheese	1 small onion, chopped
1 cup steamed broccoli florets	1 celery rib, chopped
1 cup cherry tomatoes, halved	1 small carrot, chopped
	¼ cup oil
	Juice of 1 lemon
	Salt and pepper

Toss ingredients and chill. *Makes 4–6 servings.*

NOTES: For an Italian variant, use olive oil, add pinches of basil and oregano, substitute wine vinegar for lemon juice, and ¼ cup fresh Parmesan for the mild cheese. Add a mashed clove of garlic.

For variety, use steamed zucchini in place of the broccoli and/or cucumber.

SESAME TAHINI DRESSING

¼ cup tahini (sesame paste)
1 large garlic clove, mashed

¼ cup lemon juice
Pinch of cayenne
2 teaspoons tamari

Dilute tahini, if it is very thick, with ½ cup hot water. Combine in jar with other ingredients and shake till well mixed.

TOFU-TAHINI DRESSING

¼ cup mashed tofu
¼ cup tahini (sesame paste)
½ cup carrot juice (see note)

2 tablespoons lemon juice
1–2 garlic cloves, minced
1 teaspoon tamari

Blend until smooth, or mash together until thoroughly blended.

NOTE: For carrot juice, you need a juicer. If you don't have one, you can buy bottled carrot juice in a health food store. Or grate 2 medium carrots and blend with rest of ingredients in a blender.

COOKED GREENS

A staple of cuisines as diverse as Oriental, Italian and "soul," dark leafy greens of any kind are rich in minerals, and we don't eat nearly enough of them, considering they're so easy to fix. Try to eat them at least twice a week, and try all kinds, not neglecting spinach, escarole and endive; kale, collards and the leaves of broccoli; the Italian greens rabe and arugula where available; and mustard. All of these greens cook quickly—almost instantly—wilting on contact with heat. For best results, clean them in advance, rinsing and draining thoroughly, and then cook just before serving. Don't ever boil them—sauté them or, if you are trying to restrict oil in your diet, steam them. In either case, cook them with onions or garlic to make the best of the slightly bitter taste. Sautéed onions or garlic can be quite sweet, but they are good if steamed, too. Steaming makes even garlic deliciously mild. Remember that greens shrink greatly when cooked.

GREENS, SOUTHERN STYLE

1 medium onion, chopped
¼ cup corn or peanut oil
1 pound collards or kale, thoroughly rinsed and drained

3 tablespoons vinegar
Salt and pepper
1 egg, hard-boiled and chopped

Sauté onion in oil until translucent. Add greens and sauté, stirring, until barely done. They should retain a good green color. Toss with vinegar, salt, and pepper. Garnish with chopped eggs. *Makes 4 servings.*

ITALIAN GREENS

2 garlic cloves, chopped
¼ cup olive oil
1 pound rabe, escarole,
    endive, spinach or
    arugula, washed and
    drained

Lemon juice
    (optional)
Salt
Hot pepper flakes
    (optional)

Sauté garlic in oil and add greens. Cook until barely done.
Toss in lemon juice and season with salt and pepper.   *Makes
4 servings.*

ORIENTAL GREENS

1 garlic clove, chopped
3 tablespoons sesame oil
1 slice ginger, minced
1 teaspoon or more
    tamari
1 pound kale, bok choy,
    Chinese cabbage or
    other greens

Lime juice or rice
    vinegar
Gomasio or Toasted
    Sesame Seeds
    (optional; see Index)

Sauté garlic in oil for a minute; add ginger and sauté until
garlic is turning gold. Add tamari and greens; cook barely
done. Toss with lime juice or vinegar. Garnish with Gomasio
or Toasted Sesame Seeds.   *Makes 4 servings.*

NOTE: Other greens include vegetable tops—like beet or turnip greens—if you have them. And don't forget wild greens
like mustard or dandelion, if you have the expertise to recognize them. You can also grow these "wild" greens, if you have
a garden; or you may be able to buy them fresh at produce
stands.

And don't forget to use all these greens in soups and stir-fry or other cooked vegetable dishes. The more delicate dark greens—spinach, dandelion, mustard, escarole, arugula and endive—can go into salads, too.

ZUCCHINI FRIES

A good hot hors d'oeuvre or side dish.

2 cups flour	2 eggs, beaten with 1
1 cup wheat germ	tablespoon milk
¾ cup grated Parmesan	¼ cup oil
6 small zucchini, sliced lengthwise into sticks	

Mix flour, wheat germ and Parmesan. Dip zucchini into egg, then into dry mixture. Lay sticks on a greased baking sheet, dribble oil evenly on top, and cook 15–20 minutes at 350 degrees.   *Serves 6–8 at a meal or many at a party.*

NOTE: Try it with fresh asparagus, cleaned and partly cooked by steaming. Delicious.

MARINATED VEGETABLES

Also excellent as an entrée for light summer meals. Team it with a cold cucumber soup for a heartier dinner; or serve as a side dish with grilled fish.

2 large potatoes, sliced	1 large onion, sliced thin
1½ cups green beans, broken up	2 tomatoes, sliced
1 small zucchini, sliced	Marinade (recipe follows)
1 small yellow squash, sliced	

Steam the beans and potatoes until almost tender. Add the squashes and steam until tender. Chill. Arrange on a platter with the tomatoes and onions and add marinade. Chill for an hour or two. *Serves 4.*

MARINADE

⅓ cup oil
3 tablespoons vinegar
1 large garlic clove, minced

1 teaspoon Dijon mustard
½ teaspoon dried basil
Salt and pepper

Mix and pour over the vegetables.

WHAT ABOUT LUNCH?

May we suggest: Egg and Tofu Salad, Tabbouleh sandwiches, Hummus on pita with leafy greens, and Falafel, also stuffed into pita pockets with a handful of salad greens? For the latter, you may want to carry along a little salad dressing to add to the sandwich. See Index for recipes.

Or just make a whole meal of salad, by itself or stuffed into a pita pocket—make it heartier by adding a handful of grated cheese, chopped cooked egg, or Tofu-Tahini Dressing (almost a meal in itself). Leftover Lentil Burgers make a good lunch too, as does sliced leftover Cheese and Lentil Loaf. Take soup along in a Thermos, with or without a sandwich, and a piece of fruit.

In this section are several recipes good for sandwich spreads or hors d'oeuvre.

ANYA KUCHAREVA'S EGGPLANT CAVIAR

This Eastern European dish is good on dark bread as a lunch dish or hors d'oeuvre.

1 eggplant	1 tablespoon basil
1 large onion	1 teaspoon oregano
1 garlic clove	¼ teaspoon cayenne
2 tablespoons olive oil	pepper
1 can (1 pound)	2 tablespoons tamari
tomatoes, drained	

Bake eggplant at 375 degrees for half an hour. Prick several holes in it at the start of cooking to let steam escape. Peel and chop eggplant.

Brown onion and garlic in oil. Add rest of ingredients and simmer until tomatoes and eggplant are blended. Chill and serve as a spread, or in sandwiches. *Makes 3 cups.*

BABA GHANNOUJ

A Middle Eastern eggplant dish that also makes a good light lunch or goes far as hors d'oeuvres.

1 medium eggplant, baked and peeled
2 tablespoons chopped parsley
1 large garlic clove, chopped
2 tablespoons lemon juice
2 tablespoons tahini (sesame paste)

Purée ingredients to yield a smooth paste. Let people dip in with pieces of pita bread. *Makes 1–2 cups.*

HUMMUS

2 tablespoons sesame seeds, toasted, or 2 tablespoons tahini (sesame paste)
1½ cups cooked chick-peas, or 1 15½-ounce can chick-peas, drained
½ cup chopped onion
2 garlic cloves, pressed
½ cup minced parsley
1 teaspoon oregano
2 tablespoons oil
2 tablespoons fresh lemon juice
Salt

Add toasted seeds or tahini to the chick-peas and mash. Sauté onion, garlic and herbs in the oil; add to chick-peas and blend in. Stir in lemon juice and salt to taste. Serve as an hors d'oeuvre or as a light entrée with quartered pita bread for dipping. Or use as a filling for pita sandwiches, with fresh greens or other raw vegetables. *Makes 2–3 cups.*

YEAST BREADS

Soda or quick breads rise because of a chemical interaction between the baking powder or soda and liquid ingredients in the dough. They rise quickly and are baked at once. Yeast breads rise because of the action of the yeast, which consists of many tiny live organisms, feeding on starch and sugar in the dough. Yeast breads rise slowly, and can take 6 to 8 hours to make.

Yeast comes in powder or cake form. To activate it requires mild warmth, like that needed to make yogurt. The first step in making yeast bread is to "prove" the yeast by adding it to about half a cup of the liquid in the recipe. The liquid should be heated until it feels lukewarm on your wrist; this means it is slightly warmer than your body temperature. If the yeast bubbles after sitting in a warm place in the warm liquid for a little while—up to 10 minutes—you can be sure it is good. If not, add a little sugar or honey, stir, test the warmth of the liquid, and try again. Even fine bubbles are usually a sign the yeast is good.

The second key factor in getting the bread to rise well is kneading. Unlike quick breads, yeast breads are quite sturdy and actually improve with vigorous kneading. After all ingredients are assembled and combined, the bread is turned out on a floured board and kneaded for a few minutes. Knead by flattening the dough with the hands, folding it and flattening again. It can also be slapped, dropped and pounded without ill effect.

Then the dough is set in a warm place, oiled lightly to prevent dryness, and covered with a towel. It rises for a while, usually until doubled, then is punched down and allowed to rise again. (Punch down by sticking two fingers into the middle of the dough. If the depressions fill quickly, it needs more rising time. If they stay for a bit, the dough is ready to shape.) Then it is shaped, set in pans or on a baking sheet, and allowed to rise again briefly—up to half an hour. Sometimes only two risings are called for, and the second or third is omitted.

The bread is then baked, usually in a preheated oven. It may be brushed with water, egg, milk or a combination of these to achieve a richer or shinier crust.

For best results, some wheat flour should be used in yeast bread, since wheat flour contains more gluten than other flours, and gluten is needed for the bread to rise properly. It can be unbleached or whole wheat flour. (Some flours contain no gluten at all.) Other flours can be added to vary texture and flavor. Flour is usually sifted before measuring because it eliminates lumps and adds air, making for lighter bread. Other common ingredients are egg, which makes a lighter, softer bread; milk, which makes a crumbier bread; and assorted sweeteners, cheese, fruit, nuts and other flavorings.

The following recipe is for a very basic bread, with minimal ingredients.

BASIC BREAD

1 package or 1 cake yeast	1 tablespoon sugar
2 cups warm water	1 tablespoon salt
	About 8 cups flour

Dissolve yeast in the warm water. Add sugar and salt. Add about 7 cups sifted flour and stir in thoroughly. Turn out onto floured board and knead until bread is elastic, 5–10 minutes. Oil dough lightly and place in a large bowl; cover with a clean towel; let rise in a warm place until doubled—1 to 2 hours. Punch down, turn onto floured board, and shape into two loaves, long or round. Shape loaves by flattening dough partly, then folding in both sides and ends, rather as if you were creating an envelope. Place loaves on a greased baking sheet sprinkled with corn meal. Slash tops with a knife to prevent bread tearing as it rises. Let rise again until almost doubled. Brush with cold water and set in a cold oven. Set temperature at 400 degrees and bake until crust is browned, about 45 minutes. Brush a couple of times with cold water during baking. Cool on a wire rack for a little while before cutting. *Makes 2 loaves.*

CORNELL BREAD

This bread really can serve as a meal in itself. Shape it into individual rolls if you like and pack it for snacks or lunches.

3 cups warm water	½ cup soy flour
2 cakes or packages yeast	¾ cup non-instant dry milk
2 tablespoons honey	3 teaspoons salt
7 cups flour	2 tablespoons oil
¼ cup wheat germ	

Combine water, yeast and honey. Let stand 5 minutes. Sift together flour, wheat germ, soy flour, dry milk and salt. Combine 3 cups of the flour mixture with the water and yeast mixture and stir vigorously for a minute and a half. Add oil and 3 cups more flour mixture and mix in. Turn out on board floured with remaining flour mixture and knead vigorously. Oil dough and set in a warm place to rise until doubled. Punch down and let rise again, about 20 minutes. Shape into two loaves, place in greased pans, and let rise until doubled. Bake in 350 oven about 1 hour. *Makes 2 loaves.*

DESSERTS

There's not much to add to our basic dessert philosophy: keep it simple and for special occasions. If you love raw fruit, you'll have no trouble thinking of it as dessert and keeping a bowl of seasonal fruits around for people to help themselves. Even if you're not wild about fresh fruit, try Yogurt Fruit Dessert—people love it, and it's a refreshingly light dessert. For more complicated and time-consuming desserts, use your basic pie recipe to make pies from local fruits as they come into season. If you try each one once, from strawberries in the summer through pumpkins in the fall, you'll have pie about once a month for six months of the year!

YOGURT FRUIT DESSERT

This dessert surprisingly needs no sweetener—the tartness of the lemon juice and yogurt brings out the natural sweetness of the fruit.

3 cups cut-up fruit   ½ cup Yogurt (see Index
    Juice of 1 lemon   or use plain yogurt)

Pick three or so kinds of fruit in season: in winter it might be apples, oranges and banana with a little garnish of chopped coconut; in spring, strawberries, oranges and melon; in summer, peaches, berries and melon; in fall, apples, pears and plums. Skin only the fruits that need it; scrub the rest well before cutting.

    Put in a good serving bowl, toss gently with lemon juice and then yogurt, and refrigerate until ready to serve.

TOFU CHEESECAKE

Take the plunge—you may be delighted.

2 pounds tofu, mashed
½ cup mild oil (sesame
    is good)
½ cup honey
2 teaspoon vanilla
½ teaspoon salt

¼ cup lemon juice
1 tablespoon flour
1 egg
Graham Cracker Crust
    (recipe follows)

Combine ingredients for filling in a large bowl. The egg is optional—it makes a lighter cheesecake. In a blender, mix until creamy. Pour into crust-lined 10-inch pie pan and bake at 350 degrees until golden brown, about 30 minutes. Chill before serving. Top with chilled cooked fruit, if desired. *Makes 8 servings.*

GRAHAM CRACKER CRUST

2 packages (4 ounces
    each) graham or
    other mild crackers

4 tablespoons soft
    butter or mild oil

Crumble crackers and work in the oil or butter with your fingers. Press into 10-inch pie pan.

PUMPKIN PIE

A delectable treat for fall and winter.

2 unbaked pie shells
2 cups cooked pumpkin
    (see notes)
4 eggs
1 cup yogurt

2 tablespoons molasses
4 tablespoons honey
¼ teaspoon salt
2 teaspoons cinnamon
1 teaspoon ginger

Pinch of ground
cloves
1 teaspoon vanilla
2 tablespoons brandy,
rum or bourbon
(optional)

½ cup chopped walnuts
(optional)
½ cup sliced apples
(optional)

Combine all ingredients except the walnuts and apples. Blend or beat with a rotary beater until smooth.

Pour into pie shells and, if desired, sprinkle tops of pies with nuts and apple slices. Bake at 375 degrees for 40 minutes, or until custard is firm. Serve with whipped cream or ice cream. *Two pies make 16 servings.*

NOTES: To cook the pumpkin, wash it and slice in half. Clean out seeds and pulp, scraping inside of shell clean with a spoon. Rinse and dry. Bake face down on a greased cookie sheet at 325 degrees until shell pierces easily, an hour or more. Remove skin and mash pumpkin meat. Excess can be frozen for later use.

EIGHTEEN

Recipes for Stage Three

STOCKS AND SOUPS

If you are going to eat soup often—whether it's a simple miso soup or something heartier—you'll find it a great time-saver to have soup stock on hand, though all these stocks can be made quickly. Soup stock is especially handy in the morning for a quick bowl of miso without any fuss, especially if you keep a little container of cooked noodles on hand as well. And you can use the stocks to poach vegetables or as the liquid ingredient in stews.

Kombu Stock

Do not rinse kombu unless it is dusty. Washing rinses out some of the seaweed's mineral quality. Use one piece in 2 quarts of cold water. Bring to a boil and boil for 5 minutes. Remove the kombu and let it dry out—it can be reused several times to make stock. The stock may be refrigerated and used for up to 5 days.

QUICK VEGETABLE STOCK

Cut off the top and bottom of an onion. Peel, split from top to bottom and slice into half moons. Slice in thin diagonals one small carrot. Add a half-inch chunk of daikon radish, chopped fine, if you have it, or some chopped celery. Boil in one or two quarts of water for 15–20 minutes. This stock can be made in the morning for immediate use in miso soup, or refrigerated and used throughout the week.

MUSHROOM STOCK

Boil one or two shiitake mushrooms in a quart of water for 5 minutes; turn down heat and simmer half an hour. Remove stems, cut up tops; return tops to broth. Keeps in refrigerator up to a week.

MUSHROOM-KOMBU STOCK

Soak 4 or 5 shiitake mushrooms in water for about 5 minutes. Put a piece of kombu in 2 quarts of cold water and set over high heat. Add the mushrooms and their soaking water, bring to a boil, and simmer over reduced heat 5–10 minutes. Remove kombu and set it to dry. Remove the mushrooms and reserve them for another dish, or if they are to be part of a soup right away, cut off the tough stems, slice the caps and return these to the stock. The stems may be saved to go into Scrap Stock, or onto the compost heap. Keeps up to a week.

SCRAP STOCK

If you have the time and organization to save scraps of vegetables—ends or stalks that are too tough (but have been properly cleaned), stray leaves, tops, skins or what have you—these can be refrigerated or frozen and later boiled into a Scrap Stock. Try it and see whether you like it. Things to include might be shiitake stems, broccoli stems, carrot tops, onion skins and scraps, or the center ribs from the wakame leaves. Boil for 10 minutes in several quarts of water and strain. Discard the vegetables (or put in the compost heap). Stock keeps for several days.

QUICK FISH STOCK

Boil 3 tablespoons dried bonito flakes (get them at an Oriental grocery) in 2 quarts of water for several minutes. Strain, or use with the flakes left in the stock for a heartier soup.

FISH STOCK

Boil fish scraps, heads and bones in several quarts of water for 20 minutes to half an hour. Strain off stock and allow meat and bones to cool. Remove meat from bones and save or return to stock. Discard bones or bury in the compost heap.

If you want added flavor, include stock vegetables—carrot, celery, daikon, onion—to the pot. And if you have a whole morning or day around the house, you can keep boiling the stock, adding more water, until the bones and meat dissolve into the broth. Cool and strain to remove any remaining bones. Makes a heartier, stronger-tasting broth.

MORE MISO SOUP

Nothing revolutionary here—just a review of this important food. A reminder that in macrobiotic homes, the day traditionally starts with a bowl of miso soup. A reminder too that miso is a fermented food containing enzymes that are valuable aids to digestion. These enzymes are destroyed by prolonged cooking. When miso is used as a flavoring for vegetable or bean dishes, it is just that; in cooking the enzymes are lost. But in miso soup, part of the point is to get the maximum benefit of those enzymes. So the soup should be simmered only briefly, not boiled, after the miso is added.

2 cups Mushroom or Quick Vegetable Stock (see Index)	1 leaf wakame, soaked and cut in ribbons
1 small onion, sliced in half moons	1 handful watercress or other greens, washed and drained
½ small carrot, in matchsticks	1 teaspoon tamari Cooked noodles
1 thick slice daikon, in matchsticks	1 teaspoon miso

Bring stock to a boil and add onion. Simmer 5 minutes, add carrot and daikon and simmer 5 minutes more. Add wakame and simmer 5 minutes. Add greens, tamari and noodles. Take a few spoonfuls of the liquid from pot and mix with miso in a bowl. When miso is thoroughly dissolved, return to pot and simmer for a minute.   *Makes 2 servings.*

FAVORITE BREAKFAST MISO SOUP

THE STOCK:

1 large shiitake mushroom

1 large garlic clove, minced, or ½ onion, sliced thin

1 tablespoon ginger juice (optional)

1 small carrot, chopped

1 slice daikon, chopped

Soba noodles (optional)

THE SOUP:

Greens, or 1 sheet crumbled nori, or wakame, soaked and sliced

1 teaspoon miso per cup

Boil the mushroom in 1 quart water for 5 minutes; add other stock ingredients and simmer 10–15 minutes. If desired, add soba noodles and cook until tender. Slice mushroom, discard stem and return top to soup. Stock may be used throughout the week.

To make soup, heat stock and add greens or seaweed. Simmer 5 minutes. Pour a little broth into a bowl or cup and mix with miso. Return to pot and simmer for a minute or two, stirring. Garnish, if desired, with chopped scallions or gomasio.

LENTIL SOUP

A hearty main dish or opening course.

½ cup lentils, rinsed and
    drained
1 quart Mushroom-
    Kombu Stock (see
    Index)
    Large pinch of salt

1 onion, cut in half
    moons
1 celery rib, chopped
    fine
    Tamari to taste

Cook lentils in the stock until tender, about half an hour. Add salt and vegetables (onions first), and cook until tender. If additional seasoning is desired, add tamari during last 10 minutes of cooking.

Serve as is or purée in a food mill.   *Serves 4.*

NOTES: For this soup, the mushrooms may be sliced and re-turned to the soup. If soup appears too thick, add more liquid —stock or water.

BARLEY-MUSHROOM SOUP

A hearty soup for a whole meal in itself. Serve with cooked greens and sourdough bread as side dishes.

1 cup pearl barley
1 quart or more
    Mushroom-Kombu
    Stock (see Index)
    Large pinch of sea salt

1 onion, sliced
1 carrot, sliced
1 celery rib, chopped
    Tamari

Cook the barley in the stock for 30 minutes to 1 hour—until tender. Add salt. Add vegetables and cook until tender. Add tamari near the end of the cooking. Garnish with scallions or parsley.   *Makes 6 servings.*

NOTE: For a creamier soup, add leftover cooked grain with the barley. For quicker cooking, presoak the barley for an hour and cut the vegetables into matchsticks.

ADUKI BEAN SOUP

A hearty winter soup. Serve with baked squash as a side dish, and kasha if desired.

1 cup aduki beans,
  soaked overnight
2 quarts Kombu Stock
  (see Index)
1 large pinch of sea salt

1 medium onion, sliced
1 carrot, sliced thin
1 celery rib, sliced
Tamari to taste

Add beans to kombu stock, leaving kombu in, if desired, for added digestibility. Cook until tender, about an hour. Add salt and vegetables, cook until vegetables are tender, about 20 minutes. Add tamari and simmer for a few minutes longer. *Makes 4 servings.*

NOTE: Aduki beans cook more quickly than other beans, though not as quickly as lentils or split peas. In a pinch they can be cooked simply by boiling with kombu for an hour or a little longer, without presoaking. Or they can be cooked in a pressure cooker for 30 minutes.

BLACK BEAN SOUP

A rich soup, elegant for lunch or dinner guests.

1 cup black turtle beans
1 quart Kombu Stock
  (see Index)
1 onion, sliced
1 large pinch of salt

1 carrot, sliced
Tamari (optional)
2 teaspoons mirin or
  sake per bowl

Put beans in pressure cooker with water to cover and bring to pressure. Reduce flame to low; cook 45 minutes to 1 hour. Bring pressure down and remove cover. Place beans in kombu stock with onion and salt and simmer, covered, for half an hour. Add carrots and simmer 10 minutes, adding tamari if needed. Serve, adding mirin or sake to each bowl. Garnish with chopped scallions, if desired. *Serves 4.*

NOTES: To make the beans more nutritious and digestible, soak them overnight, discard soaking water, and cook them slowly in kombu stock instead of pressure cooking. They should cook up to 2 hours. This will require more liquid; if you like, simply start with 2 or 3 quarts water and leave the kombu in for the duration of cooking.

BONITO NOODLE SOUP

A good answer to chicken noodle anytime.

1 strip kombu	10–12 snow pea pods
4–5 shiitake mushrooms, soaked	1 carrot, sliced thin
	¼ pound udon noodles, cooked
1 small package (about 2 ounces) bonito flakes	Roasted nori, daikon radish, or chopped scallions
Tamari	

Make stock with 1 quart water, kombu, shiitakes and bonito, simmered 5–7 minutes. Strain and add tamari to taste.

Parboil snow pea pods that have been cleaned (ends pinched off and strings, if any, removed) and carrots. Add these and the noodles to the stock and simmer briefly. Garnish with roasted nori, crumbled or snipped into matchsticks using scissors, or with daikon cut into matchsticks, or with scallions. *Serves 4.*

NOTES: This recipe came from Susan Ingram, a macrobiotics teacher, who explains that it's important to use a pungent-tasting garnish to balance the noodles and aid digestion. Hence the daikon or scallion; ginger may also be used.

PUMPKIN SOUP

A hearty and inexpensive winter meal. Winter squash (butternut, acorn) may be substituted. The fried onion and the sesame seeds help balance the sweetness of the pumpkin.

1 medium onion, chopped	Fresh ginger, grated
	Parsley
1 cup cooked pumpkin (see notes)	Gomasio
	Salt
Oil	
Flour	
1 quart hot Quick Vegetable Stock or other stock (see Index)	

Sauté the onion and pumpkin in a little oil. Set to boil in stock, then turn down to a simmer. Using a couple of tablespoons of oil, a tablespoon of flour and a cup of stock, make a light sauce, like a white sauce. Set aside. Purée the pumpkin and onion in a blender or food mill, and return to stock. Add the sauce, stirring to blend, and let simmer 5 minutes more. Garnish with grated ginger and parsley, and season to taste with gomasio. *Makes 6 servings.*

NOTES: To cook a fresh pumpkin, cut off the top, scrape out the seeds and strings, and wash all over. Cut in half, and put face down on a greased cookie sheet. Let bake at 350 degrees for half an hour, until soft. The unused portion may be frozen for soups or pies. Seeds may be saved for roasting or planting.

By the way, a pumpkin is a pretty sturdy fruit, and may be

used as a jack-o-lantern first, then washed and baked. Just be sure to remove any wax from the inside.

HOT AND SOUR SOUP

This is not really a macrobiotic soup, because of the egg and the richness of the dish, but totally delicious. It is included here because of its use of such macrobiotic ingredients as the shiitake and kudzu. You can always omit the egg and the cayenne pepper for a more truly macrobiotic meal.

This soup is an elegant party dish, and rich enough to be a meal in itself.

Handful of dried daylily buds (from an Oriental grocery)	2 tablespoons mirin
	4 tablespoons brown rice vinegar
1 dried "wood ear," broken into pieces (Oriental grocery)	2 tablespoons tamari
	Salt
	Cayenne pepper
Sliced cooked shiitake mushrooms from stock	⅛ cup kudzu, dissolved in ⅓ cup water
1 pound tofu, cut into strips	1 egg, beaten
	1 bunch chopped scallions
1 quart Mushroom Stock (see Index)	

Simmer the lily buds, wood ear fungus, shiitake mushrooms and tofu in the stock about 15 minutes. Add mirin, vinegar and tamari, and simmer 15 minutes more. Taste, and correct seasoning, adding salt and more tamari if needed, plus cayenne pepper for hotness if needed. Add kudzu-water mixture, stirring constantly to blend in. Just before serving, stir in egg and remove from heat at once. Garnish with scallions. *Serves 4.*

NOTE: For added taste and texture interest, add thin slices of daikon radish and carrot cut in half moons; put them in at the same time as the tofu. Chopped leafy greens (spinach, Chinese cabbage, escarole) may be added after the kudzu.

ONION SOUP WITH FU ROUNDS

The old Parisian standby in macrobiotic guise. A festive dish for company from Susan Ingram's kitchen.

6–8 onions, sliced into half-moons	Tamari (optional)
Sesame oil	1 fu round per person, soaked in water
Kombu	Watercress or parsley
2 ounces bonito flakes	
2 tablespoons white miso	

Sauté onions in sesame oil to a deep golden color. Create a broth with 2 quarts water, the kombu and bonito flakes; strain. Cook the onions in the broth, simmering an hour or more. Dilute the miso with a little broth and add near end of cooking. Add tamari if desired and simmer a few minutes more. Garnish with fu rounds, soaked until soft, or with chopped cress or parsley. *Makes 6–8 servings.*

NOTES: For a touch of Les Halles, pour the onion soup into an oven-proof dish near the end of cooking. Spread each fu round with a little white miso and float them in the broth. Slip under the broiler for a minute or two to melt the miso for a cheese effect.

If you have trouble finding fu rounds, toasted rounds or triangles of sourdough bread may be used.

WATERCRESS SOUP

1 cup cooked leftover
  grain
1 quart Quick Vegetable
  Stock (see Index)
1 tablespoon salt

1 small onion, cut into
  half-moon slices
3 handfuls of chopped
  cleaned watercress
Tamari (optional)

Boil the cooked grain in the stock with salt until it begins to
turn creamy. Then add onion and cook 10 minutes. Add watercress, and tamari if desired. Cook until watercress is just
tender. If a velvety texture is desired, cream the soup in a
blender. *Makes 6 servings.*

MILLET SOUP

1 cup millet
1 tablespoon oil
1 quart Mushroom-
  Kombu Stock (see
  Index)
2 onions, chopped
1 large carrot, cut into
  matchsticks

¼ head cabbage, sliced
  fine
Sea salt
Chopped watercress
  or scallions

Roast the millet in the oil over medium flame, stirring to
brown it gently. Add to boiling stock, and cook 30 minutes.
Add vegetables and cook, covered, for 20 minutes. Season
with salt to taste and cook 5 minutes.

Garnish with chopped cress or scallions if desired. *Makes
6 servings.*

NOTE: Instead of cabbage, try escarole, kale or other dark
green vegetable. The alkaline millet and the bitter greens
make a good blend of tastes and are a very healthy dish.

MACROBIOTIC MINESTRONE

1 quart Mushroom
   Stock (see Index)
½ cup split peas, rinsed
   and drained
1 carrot, sliced thin
1 onion, sliced thin
1 bay leaf
1 cup macaroni
1 small summer squash,
   sliced

2 celery ribs, chopped
½ cup cooked beans or
   garbanzos
½ cup cooked leftover
   grain (optional)
1 teaspoon salt
1 cup shredded cabbage

Bring stock to a boil with the split peas, carrot, onion and bay leaf; reduce heat and simmer about 45 minutes. Meanwhile, cook the macaroni and chop the other vegetables. When the split peas are tender, add squash, celery, beans, macaroni, cooked grain if used, and salt. Cook 5 minutes, add the cabbage, and cook 5 minutes more.   *About 6–8 servings.*

NOTES: The bay leaf is a concession to Italian cooking, not a regular part of macrobiotic cuisine.

   The cooked leftover grain may be added to the stock earlier, with the split peas, to impart a rich, creamy texture to the soup. This is also a good soup for using up any kind of leftover beans.

VEGETABLE AND BEAN ENTRÉES

Some of these dishes are elegant enough to be used for entertaining, but none is very complicated. And don't forget basic stir-fry, with tofu or nuts or just plain, introduced in Stage One.

BROILED TOFU

This is about the quickest protein dish there is. Good for speedy suppers, and especially handy if you are cooking meat for some of the diners and want a non-meat entrée for the others.

1-inch chunk of ginger	½ pound tofu, sliced ¼-
1 tablespoon tamari	inch thick
1 teaspoon sesame oil	
1 tablespoon lemon juice (optional)	

Rinse and grate the ginger, and squeeze out juice. Mix juice with tamari and oil, and dilute with 1 part water to 2 parts sauce. Add lemon juice, if desired. Pour over tofu. Broil 5–7 minutes. Garnish with chopped scallions or parsley, if desired. *Serves 2.*

"CHEESE" TOFU

White miso	Chopped scallions or
½ pound tofu, sliced	parsley

Mix several tablespoons of miso and water into a rich cream. Pour over tofu and broil 5 minutes for a cheesy effect. Garnish with chopped scallions or parsley.　*Serves 2.*

STUFFED SQUASH

A good solution for large squashes. The filling here is enough for the halves of one large summer or winter squash.

THE FILLING:

2 tablespoons tamari	6 large mushrooms, chopped
2 tablespoons mirin	
½ cup crumbled tempeh	1 small carrot, chopped
2 cups cooked grain	Oil
1 cup minced onion	¼ cup white miso
¼ cup chopped celery	

Mix the tamari, mirin and ½ cup water; pour over the tempeh and set aside to marinate. If cooked grain is needed (unless you have leftovers), set it to boil. Sauté the vegetables in oil.

After the tempeh has marinated half an hour, set it to simmer in the pan used to cook the vegetables, adding water if needed. Simmer half an hour. Mix with the grain and vegetables.

Fill the halves of a large squash, split and seeded, with the mixture. Top with white miso mixed with water to form a thick cream. Bake in a 375-degree oven for 20 minutes. *Makes 4 servings.*

NOTES: Some people prefer to cook the squash meat in with the rest of the filling. If this is your preference, first remove the squash meat from the shell. To do this for a summer squash, simply scoop out with a spoon or knife. For a winter squash, split and seed it and bake face down on a greased cookie sheet in a 350-degree oven for about 20 minutes.

Next, proceed to make the filling, chopping the squash fairly fine and mixing in with the vegetables during sautéing.

Some people find they don't like the taste of the white miso. If you find this is the case, you can omit it. You may also substitute a paste made from tofu blended with water and lemon juice—about ¼ cake of tofu, juice of 1 lemon and a little water—or with tahini diluted with water and lemon juice.

TEMPEH STEW

A good summer stew. Serve with cooked greens and sourdough bread on the side.

12–16 baby onions or shallots	Ginger juice
½–¾ pound tempeh, cut into squares	2 small yellow squashes, cut into chunks
Heaping tablespoon of white miso	¼ pound green beans

Put onions in boiling water to cover. Reduce heat and simmer for 5 minutes. Add tempeh and miso, diluted with water, and the juice of a 1-inch chunk of ginger. Cook half an hour. Add the squash and the green beans, and cook until beans are tender.   *Makes 3–4 servings.*

NOTE: This dish may be "winterized" by substituting carrots, cauliflower and broccoli for the squash and beans.

SUKIYAKI

A traditional favorite, skillet-cooked vegetables, in a little broth. A wonderful dish for company; bring it to the table and let people help themselves. Cut vegetables to give pleasing, delicate shapes; select them for a beautiful mixture of colors. Cook just long enough to get a pleasing texture; longer-cooking vegetables may be parboiled before adding to the broth. Serve in the traditional style with rice and side dishes of condiments for dipping; or incorporate one condiment into the broth for a less fancy dish.

THE VEGETABLES:
  Broccoli florets
  Carrot slices
  Yellow squash in half moons
  Shallots or small onions, halved
  Chinese cabbage, shredded
  Celery, sliced
  Watercress, cleaned and chopped
  Bean sprouts

THE BROTH:
  4 parts water to 1 part tamari

CONDIMENTS:
  Tamari and citrus juice
  White miso and citrus juice
  Mirin and ginger juice

Arrange vegetables beautifully; add enough broth to simmer briefly without burning. Cook quickly over medium-high heat without covering. Serve with small dishes of condiments.

NOTE: Other vegetables could include onions in half moons, snow peas, cauliflower and green beans. Other ingredients, for a fancy meal, could include tofu, precooked noodles, precooked fish or scallops.

SUSHI

For this recipe you need at least one sushi mat, available at Oriental groceries.

1 thin strip tempeh per person
Cooked rice
Carrot strips
Cucumber strips

1 sheet nori per person
Brown rice vinegar, or umeboshi paste, diluted with water

THE MARINADE:

1 part tamari to 2 parts water, plus 1 teaspoon mirin per cup

Marinate the tempeh in enough marinade to cover for a couple of hours and then simmer in the marinade for 45 minutes, adding water if necessary. Cook the rice in a pressure cooker, making it wetter and softer than usual by using more water and cooking a little longer than usual. Cut the vegetables into very thin strips, allowing 1 long strip or equivalent per nori roll. Toast the nori sheets, preferably over an open flame, or over an electric burner set on high, by passing gently over the heat source until the nori changes color.

When all ingredients are ready, lay a nori sheet on the sushi mat. Its longest sides should be running in the same direction as the sticks of the mat.

Stir enough brown rice vinegar or diluted umeboshi paste through the rice to give it a tart flavor. Spread a layer of rice on the nori, leaving half an inch on the long sides. Lay filling, 1 strip of each vegetable and 1 strip of tempeh, on top lengthwise.

Roll up sushi mat to form nori roll, making sure the seam

of the nori roll is closed. Roll the closed sushi mat back and forth a few times to pack and seal the nori roll.

With a wetted knife, gently cut the roll in half with a sawing motion and trim off ends, cleaning and wetting knife before each cut. Slice each half in thirds and arrange sushi slices on a plate. *Allow 1 roll per person, or less for hors d'oeuvres.*

TOFU STEW

1 shiitake mushroom	1 celery rib, sliced
2 small onions, cut in half-moons	1 pound tofu, cut into chunks
1 carrot, sliced thin	Kudzu
6 fresh mushrooms, sliced	Tamari

Boil the shiitake mushroom 5–7 minutes in 1 quart water. Add onions and boil 5 minutes. Add carrots, mushrooms, celery and tofu. Dissolve a little kudzu in cold water and add to stew to thicken. Season with tamari. Slice shiitake mushroom and return to stew. *Makes 4 servings.*

PIROGI

Pies and turnovers of various kinds are a staple dish in most cuisines—one of the original "fast" foods. They travel well and can be eaten as finger food. Various kinds of dough, including yeast and sourdoughs, as well as egg-noodle doughs, are used.

THE DOUGH:

2 cups flour, unbleached white or whole wheat pastry	Salt
	⅓–½ cup oil
	Ice water

THE FILLING:

2 cups finely chopped sautéed vegetables	1 cup leftover cooked grain
Nuts (optional)	Finely chopped cooked fish or shrimp (optional)
Crumbled tofu (optional)	

Sift flour and salt. Blend in oil with fingers to a coarse consistency. Add water to form dough. Knead on a floured board until elastic. Chill.

For the filling, prepare the vegetables—carrots, onions, cabbage, daikon, scallions or watercress are some possibilities. Include chopped nuts if you like. Mix with the cooked grain and set aside. For a fancier effect, add tofu or fish.

Roll the dough out fairly thin, almost as for noodles, a little at a time, cutting into 3- or 4-inch rounds. Put a couple of tablespoons of filling in each pirogi cutout, fold over and seal.

Chill thoroughly before cooking. Deep fry, or brush with oil and bake at 350 degrees on a greased cookie sheet until nicely browned. *Makes 6–8 servings.*

NOTE: Pastry flour is lower in gluten than all-purpose flour and makes a lighter crust. Buy it at the health-food store.

WONTONS:

Use the Pirogi recipe, but make the dumplings smaller. Cook in soup, deep fry, or bake. The fried or baked wontons may also be topped with a white sauce made of flour, oil and vegetable stock, seasoned with tamari, mirin, or a little white miso.

MILLET-VEGETABLE CASSEROLE

1 cup millet	½ acorn squash, sliced
1 carrot, sliced	1 tablespoon oil
1 medium onion, sliced	2 tablespoons tamari

Roast the millet in a heavy pan. Set aside. Sauté the vegetables in oil. Put millet, vegetables, tamari and 3 cups water in pressure cooker. Bring to pressure, cook 20 minutes, and let pressure come down slowly. *Makes 2–3 servings.*

NOTES: Instead of pressure cooking, you can bake in a covered ovenproof dish 40 minutes at 325 degrees, or until grain is tender and water is more or less absorbed.

For a fancier dish, use more vegetables, including bean sprouts, or add nuts or chunks of tofu.

CAULIFLOWER BAKE

An elegant entrée taught by Susan Ingram. Good for entertaining. Serve with pilaf and a salad.

1 head cauliflower	⅓ cup pastry flour
⅓ cup tahini (sesame paste)	⅓ cup water
	1 tablespoon tamari

Clean cauliflower head, removing leaves and stem, and boil, whole, in salted water for 20 minutes. Mix remaining ingredients. Place cauliflower in a lightly greased pan and pour sauce over it. Bake at 350 degrees for half an hour, until crust is formed. Cut cauliflower into quarters. *Makes 4 servings.*

NOTE: Other sauces can be made with combinations of tofu and white miso, mashed together with enough water to dilute; white miso and lemon juice; or sesame paste (tahini) with any of these. Whatever the combination, add some pastry flour to insure that the sauce will adhere to the cauliflower. Add water to dilute as needed.

TOFU KEBABS

A good dish for cookouts.

Carrot chunks	Shiitake mushrooms
Squash chunks	Tofu chunks
Broccoli florets	Kudzu Sauce (recipe
Onion chunks	follows)

Parboil vegetables, except onions and mushrooms. Leave onions raw. Mushrooms should be cooked 45 minutes, with kombu, in enough water to cover, and then quartered. Thread vegetables and tofu on skewers. Baste with sauce and cook briefly under broiler or over charcoal.

KUDZU SAUCE

1–2 tablespoons kudzu	Dash of tamari
1 cup orange juice	Ginger juice
1 teaspoon mirin	

Dissolve kudzu in 1 cup cold water. Heat, stirring constantly, until translucent. Mix in other ingredients and pour over kebabs.

TOFU LASAGNE

The macrobiotic version. If this is too exotic, remember, you can still mix tofu into a more conventional lasagne. It won't be macrobiotic, but it's a step in that direction.

1 medium zucchini,
  sliced
1 medium onion,
  sliced
  Oil
8–10 whole lasagne
  noodles, cooked
1 cup parboiled
  broccoli florets

Lemon juice
1½ pounds tofu,
  crumbled
2 tablespoons tahini
2 tablespoons white
  miso
1 tablespoon tamari

Sauté zucchini and onions in oil. Drain off excess liquid. Line bottom of a greased 9-inch baking pan with noodles. Top with a layer of zucchini, onions and broccoli. Sprinkle with lemon juice.

Top with a layer of tofu, up to 1 pound. Top with a layer of noodles. Mix remaining tofu into a creamy sauce with tahini, miso, tamari and ½ cup water or more, and spread over the noodles. Bake in a 350-degree oven for 30 minutes. *Makes 4 servings.*

BASIC BEANS

This recipe can be used to prepare any beans. The aduki beans are the most digestible, and in a pinch may be cooked without soaking overnight. But soaked beans are best. Remember, discard the soaking liquid and start out with fresh water (or stock) to cook the beans. One of the reasons that soaked beans are more digestible is that indigestible fats begin to break down during the soaking process and are dissolved out of the bean and into the soaking liquid. To cook with the soaking liquid defeats part of the purpose of soaking. Small amounts of minerals may be lost in soaking, but beans are sufficiently high in minerals so that it doesn't matter.

1 strip kombu
1 celery rib, sliced

1 large onion, quartered
1 carrot, cut into chunks

½ cup aduki beans, or 1   1 tablespoon salt
   cup larger beans,   Tamari or mirin
   cleaned and soaked   Gomasio (optional)

Layer vegetables in a heavy saucepan, putting kombu on
bottom, then celery, onions and carrots, then the beans. Add
water to cover, cover pot, and bring to a boil. After 15 minutes, add ½ cup of cold water to "shock" the beans and
hasten cooking.

Add salt when beans have cooked another half hour. Cook
20 minutes longer, or until beans are tender. Taste and correct seasoning with tamari or mirin if beans seem too bland.
Garnish with gomasio if desired.   *Makes 3–4 servings.*

BASIC BEANS AND RICE

Start the bean recipe with an extra 2–3 cups water. When you
add the salt, add 1 cup of rice. Cover and cook until tender,
adding extra water if needed to prevent burning.

GRAIN DISHES

Remember that grains should ideally constitute 50 percent of each meal. That means that a cooked grain dish will be eaten alongside an entrée that doesn't already have grain in it, or eaten in addition to soup and salad, or included in soup for a simple one-pot meal.

Grains may be cooked whole grains, or cooked grain products, from kasha, couscous and bulgur wheat to whole wheat noodles, soba noodles and bread.

RICE BALLS

Easy to make, rice balls are a mainstay of macrobiotic lunch bags. They are a handy way to use up leftover grain; handy also because the combination of nori and umeboshi helps preserve the rice, even without refrigeration, for several days. And they are tasty and nutritious.

½ nori sheet per ball   ¼ umeboshi plum per
    About ½ cup cooked   ball
      rice per ball

The rice should be pressure-cooked so that it will be wet and sticky. Use more water and cook it longer than usual. Allow it to cool, while toasting the nori sheets. Each ball needs half a nori sheet, and each half sheet must be cut in half again.

Take a good handful—half a cup or so—of the cooked rice and shape it into a flattened ball, using one hand to hold the rice and the other to turn, squeeze and shape it. When the rice is in a firm cake, indent one side with a fingertip and press the umeboshi into the center of the ball. Plug the indentation with a little rice, and wrap the ball in the nori, using one quarter sheet for each side of the ball. The corners of the nori should fit together so that it completely covers the ball. One rice ball makes a light lunch or a good snack.

NOTES: You can use leftover grains in rice balls, too, but if they are dried out you will need to add a little water and let them sit and absorb it for half an hour or so, otherwise the balls will be hard to handle.

Both nori and umeboshi plums are said to aid digestion. Umeboshi has been called the "Alka-Seltzer of the Orient." Nori is higher in B vitamins than other sea vegetables, which may be why it is credited with helping to regulate the digestion. It may be a form of nourishment for healthy intestinal flora.

SESAME NOODLES

A rich dish, but simple to make.

Soba noodles	Oil
Tahini (sesame paste)	Roasted sesame seeds
Tamari	(optional)
Grated ginger	

Cook desired quantity of noodles. Dissolve the sesame butter (tahini) in water to form a thick sauce and add tamari. Sauté the ginger in a little oil and add noodles to the pan, tossing well. Stir the sauce through the noodles, tossing well over low heat. Add roasted seeds if desired. Serve hot or cold.

NOTE: The addition of cooked vegetables makes this a great entrée or party buffet dish. To the noodles and sesame sauce, add cooked string beans, squash, broccoli or mushrooms; toss and serve hot or cold.

KASHA WITH VEGETABLE GRAVY

2 cups kasha
2 tablespoons oil
Salt
1 large onion, chopped
1 cup shredded cabbage
2 large carrots, cut into matchsticks

3 shiitake mushrooms, soaked
½ cup flour
2 tablespoons tamari
1 tablespoon tahini (sesame paste)

Roast the kasha with 1 tablespoon of the oil in a heavy pan, stirring, until golden brown. Cool, then add 5–6 cups water and a pinch of salt. Bring to boil, and simmer covered over a low flame for 5 minutes. Turn off heat and allow to steam, covered.

Sauté the vegetables in 1 tablespoon oil. Dry roast the flour lightly in a saucepan; cool and add 2 cups water. Bring to a boil, stirring. Add the tamari, sesame butter and vegetables, and cook, stirring constantly, for several minutes.

Lay the kasha in a greased oven-proof dish and pour vegetable gravy over it. Bake at 300 degrees for half an hour. *Makes 4–6 servings.*

CABBAGE ROLLS

Parboiled cabbage leaves
Kasha with Vegetable Gravy (above)

Kombu, soaked in 1 cup water
White miso (optional)

Use large leaves with the base of the stem cut out for ease in folding.

Fill each leaf with several tablespoons of the kasha, topped with vegetable gravy. Roll up and secure with toothpicks. Lay kombu in baking dish and cover with soaking water. Place cabbage rolls in dish. If desired, top with a white miso-water cream sauce. Or extra Vegetable Gravy may be set aside for a topping. Bake at 350 degrees for 25–30 minutes. *Allow 2 per person.*

BOILED RICE WITH CORN

A lighter dish for summer.

1 cup rice	Pinch of sea salt
2 cups fresh corn kernels	

Wash and dry-roast rice in a heavy pan over medium-high heat. Long- and medium-grain rice may be used for this warm-weather meal. When rice is three quarters dry, add corn and salt. Add 2 cups cold water. Bring to boil, reduce heat, and boil, covered, until water is absorbed and rice is tender. *Makes 6 servings.*

FRIED RICE

Two great ways to use leftover rice.

SUMMER RICE:
    Summer squash, chopped fine
    Chinese cabbage, shredded
    Bean sprouts or snow peas
    Oil
    Cooked rice
    Tamari
    Scallions, chopped, for garnish

WINTER RICE:
    Onions, cut into half moons
    Carrots, chopped fine
    Cabbage, shredded
    Oil
    Cooked rice
    Tamari
    Daikon, shredded, for garnish
    Sunflower seeds, roasted

Allow ¼ to ½ cup vegetables per cup of rice. Sauté the vegetables lightly in oil and cover with a "lid" of rice. Add a little water; when it boils, turn down heat and let the rice steam until hot. Do not use a pot lid, the color of the vegetables will be better without it. Add tamari near the end of cooking. Garnish summer rice with scallions. Garnish winter rice with grated daikon radish and/or sunflower seeds, rinsed and then dry-roasted in a heavy skillet.

SALADS, SIDE DISHES
AND PICKLES

Some ideas about side dishes, including salads and dressings, to add interest and nutritional value to your meals. Don't hesitate to invent your own side dishes from any combination of land or sea vegetables that pleases you.

Vegetables may be boiled, parboiled, baked, sautéed, steamed or pressed. Heat, pressure and time are the factors that "cook" our vegetables, making them more digestible. In hottest weather, they may be eaten raw or in a quick-pressed day pickle, where pressure and a little time but no heat are used to "cook" the dish.

In winter, don't forget whole or halved winter squashes, simply baked. Mix spaghetti squash with noodles and eat as a main or side dish. Eat root vegetables and ground vegetables, not forgetting parsnips and turnips and members of the cabbage family as well as the squashes.

In summer, eat the lighter vegetables, including summer squashes, leafy greens, red radishes, cucumbers, green beans and sprouts.

In dressings, citrus juice is used mostly in hot weather, but brown rice vinegar can be used anytime. Brown rice vinegar is much milder than the commercial vinegars and should be used whenever vinegar is called for. Keep in mind in using oil that many macrobiotics teachers recommend limiting oil intake to 2 tablespoons a day. Most beginners probably will use more, but it is a measure to gauge your oil use by.

SKILLET SALAD

1 medium onion, cut into half-moons	Tamari
1 yellow squash, cut into half-moons	Brown rice vinegar
2 cups greens, rinsed and chopped	Gomasio (see Index) or Wakame-Sesame Condiment (see Index)
Oil	

Sauté vegetables lightly in oil in a wok or skillet—onions first, greens last. Add a little tamari (1 teaspoon) with the greens. Toss with vinegar in a ceramic or glass dish. Serve warm or cooled with gomasio or wakame-sesame condiment. *Makes 3–4 servings.*

QUICK PICKLE

2–3 small cucumbers, sliced thin	½ cup tamari
2–3 red radishes, sliced thin	2 tablespoons brown rice vinegar
3 tablespoons chopped daikon	

Put vegetables in salad press, add tamari, vinegar and 1 cup water, mix, and screw down press. Let sit for an hour or more. Drain off excess liquid and serve. *Makes 4 or more servings.*

NOTE: For this and other quick-pressed salad dishes, the small plastic salad presses available in department stores or kitchen supply stores are fine. If you don't have one of these, you can use a ceramic bowl, a plate and a weight (a gallon jug of water will do). Layer vegetables in the dish, cover with a plate and put the weight on the plate. A dish with straight sides will work best, pressing most evenly.

GOMASIO

Use as a table condiment instead of salt. May be used in cooking too.

½ teaspoon salt
3 tablespoons sesame
    seeds

Heat salt in heavy skillet until it smells faintly of chlorine. Add seeds and roast until golden brown, stirring to prevent burning. If seeds pop, turn down heat a little, cover, and shake like popcorn. When done, grind to fine powder using a suribachi mortar and pestle. Store in refrigerator.

WAKAME-SESAME CONDIMENT

An easy way to get a little seaweed into the diet. Use at table as you would gomasio, on soups, salads and main dishes.

3–4 strips wakame   Roasted sesame seeds

Toast wakame in 375-degree oven on baking sheet until almost charred. Grind with seeds in suribachi mortar and pestle: ½ wakame to ½ seeds, or ¼ wakame to ¾ seeds.

PRESSED SALAD

A refreshing summer salad.

Cucumbers, sliced thin	Red radish, in thin half-moons
Iceberg lettuce, sliced thin	Grated carrot
Romaine lettuce, sliced thin	Salt
	Umeboshi Dressing (recipe follows)

Rub cucumber rinds with salt to draw out bitterness before slicing. Press vegetables, sprinkled with salt, in salad press for as little as 45 minutes or as long as overnight. Use a makeshift press if necessary. When done, rinse with cool water to remove salt, and squeeze gently with hands to remove excess liquid. Chill if desired. Serve with dressing.

NOTES: The technique of rubbing the cucumber ends to remove bitterness is a good one to use in general whenever you have a cucumber recipe. Slice off the ends, sprinkle with salt, and rub the sliced surfaces together until a foam appears. Rinse it off.

In this salad, parboiled vegetables—cauliflower, broccoli, corn, snow peas—may also be used.

UMEBOSHI DRESSING

3 umeboshi plums	2 tablespoons mirin
3 tablespoons water	Dash of tamari
Juice of 1 lemon	2–3 chopped scallions

Blend or mash in a suribachi.

THREE-BEAN SALAD

½ cup chick-peas, soaked
  overnight
½ cup kidney beans,
  soaked overnight
  Handful of green
  beans

Kombu
Sea salt
Parsley Umeboshi
  Dressing (recipe
  follows)

Cook the beans separately. The dried beans should be boiled or pressure-cooked with kombu.

Boil the green beans until just tender. Cut into half-inch pieces and toss with the other beans, the salt and the dressing. *Makes 6 servings.*

PARSLEY UMEBOSHI DRESSING

3–4 umeboshi plums
  1 teaspoon umeboshi
  juice
¼ cup brown rice
  vinegar

1 tablespoon mirin
½ cup chopped parsley

Mash plums with liquids. Stir in parsley.

BOILED VEGETABLE SALAD

  Salt
1 yellow squash, cut
  into chunks
1 cup cauliflower florets

1 cup broccoli florets
  White Miso Dressing
  (recipe follows)

Bring a quart of water to boil with a pinch of salt. Boil each vegetable separately without putting on lid and remove while still brilliant colored. (Salt and not covering them help preserve color.) Vegetables should be tender if squeezed gently.

Stop cooking action by rinsing under cold water. Serve cold with dressing. *Makes 4–6 servings.*

NOTE: For a winter version, use carrots instead of squash.

WHITE MISO DRESSING

1 tablespoon white miso
  Juice of 1 lemon, or ¼
    cup vinegar

Mix with water to a creamy texture and toss lightly into vegetables.

BOILED GREEN SALAD WITH SPROUTS

A colander of kale or
  collard greens,
  washed
Salt
1 or 2 handfuls of mung
  bean sprouts

1 cucumber
  Mirin Dressing
    (recipe follows)

Boil greens till stems are tender in a pot of water with a pinch of salt.

Parboil sprouts by dunking them in the boiling water, using a sieve or colander. Rinse under cool water.

Slice off ends of cucumber and draw out bitterness, using salt.

Chop greens, slice cucumbers and mix with sprouts. Toss with dressing. *Makes 4 servings.*

MIRIN DRESSING

1 tablespoon mirin	Dash of tamari
¼ cup brown rice vinegar	

Mix in bowl and toss with vegetables.

HIZIKI WITH CARROTS AND ONIONS

Macrobiotics teachers recommend hiziki for its high mineral content.

Small handful of hiziki	1 small carrot, cut into
1 onion, sliced into half moons	matchsticks
1 teaspoon oil	Tamari

Rinse the hiziki. Soak 5–7 minutes in water. Save the soaking water. Cut up the seaweed.

Sauté onions in oil. Add hiziki. Sauté, add carrots, and sauté again. Add water and simmer 45 minutes to an hour. Cook longer in winter, less in summer. After 20 minutes, add a little tamari—not much, for the hiziki itself is high in minerals and has a salty taste.   *Makes 3–4 servings.*

NOTES: If water doesn't evaporate, take off lid. Add more water if needed.

Other land vegetables may be added; also roasted sesame seeds, shiitake, tofu or deep-fried tofu (winter).

In summer, cold cooked hiziki may be mixed with cucumber, lettuce and radishes for a salad.

VEGETABLE SAUTÉ

A good side dish. Add little chunks of tofu and thinly sliced onions for a more substantial stir-fry. Vary by using tamari instead of salt or by adding other vegetables.

Carrots, finely chopped	Watercress, rinsed and chopped
Chinese cabbage, shredded	Oil
	Salt

Sauté vegetables (carrots first, watercress last) in a little oil, adding salt with each vegetable.

BREAD

Sourdough bread is preferred to yeast breads in macrobiotic cooking because it is more digestible. It is made from a starter that takes the place of commercial yeast. The starter consists of a flour-water base that is allowed to ferment from the yeast organisms in the air. If you have no success in creating your own starter, commercial starters can be obtained.

SOURDOUGH BREAD

1 cup sourdough starter   3 cups flour
   (recipe follows)   Large pinch of salt
1 cup or more
   lukewarm water

Mix ingredients thoroughly and place in an oiled bowl. Oil top of dough lightly and cover bowl with a damp towel. Place in a warm spot for 8–24 hours, checking periodically for activity. Turn dough out on a lightly floured board, knead thoroughly (at least 5 minutes), and return to bowl. Let rise until almost doubled. Punch down, knead again, and shape into loaf, which may be set in a greased pan or on a baking sheet. Let rise again for an hour. Slash top with a sharp knife. Bake in a 350-degree oven until bread is nicely browned, 45 minutes to an hour.

SOURDOUGH STARTER

Set 1 cup flour and 1 cup warm water, mixed together with any leftover grain you happen to have handy, out on a counter overnight. It may be lightly covered with a sushi mat or napkin. After 24 hours, stir to see if you have bubbles, indicating that the starter is "live." If not, move to a slightly warmer place, like the top of the stove, and add a little honey or barley malt. Wait 6–8 hours and check again.

NOTE: Working with sourdough that does not include any yeast is rather like working with the heavier flours (rye, for instance). The dough can be so heavy that you're sure you've done something wrong. You haven't. Even when it's baked it will be very heavy, and should be sliced very thin and toasted if you like. Also, in working with the dough you may find it very sticky. There's no real remedy except to keep flouring the board and your hands and try to keep on top of the situation.

If you want to lighten the bread a bit, you can incorporate 1 tablespoon yeast. Simply add yeast to the starter before adding other ingredients, and stir in well. (This is not a macrobiotic method, but a conventional sourdough, when yeast is used.)

DESSERTS

For anyone who has the idea that macrobiotics is an ascetic
way of life, the dessert section may be reassuring. Experiment with your favorite fruits, using kanten to gel them, or
kudzu for sauces and puddings—even pies. Besides these
recipes, don't forget stewed and baked fruits. In summer the
choice is abundant. In winter, use dried fruits occasionally in
stewing, or for puddings or pies.

APPLESAUCE

6 apples
  Pinch of salt

Wash and quarter apples; don't core them. Boil in 1 cup
water with salt. Strain out excess juice and run apples
through food mill to strain out seeds and skins.   *Makes 4–6
servings.*

NOTES: Stayman, Winesap and Rome Beauty apples are good
for sauce. Use pears, too, with the apples or by themselves.

Try adding raisins too, during cooking or after. If they are
cooked and milled with the apples, you will get the flavor
without the whole raisins. If you want whole raisins, add
them with a little of the excess juice to the milled apples and
return to the stove for a little extra cooking to plump the
raisins. Add a squeeze of lemon juice during cooking for a
tarter taste.

Save the excess juice for drinking, or add it to bancha tea
for a special occasion, or use it in pumpkin soup.

If you don't have a food mill, you can use a blender, food
processor or potato masher, followed by an egg beater. But

you will have to skin and core the apples before cooking, losing some nutritive value. *Makes 6–8 servings.*

BERRIES WITH KANTEN

Would you believe macrobiotic Jell-O?

3 cups apple juice
  Pinch of salt
1 bar kanten (agar-agar)

3 cups fresh berries,
  cleaned and washed

Heat apple juice with salt and kanten to dissolve, then simmer 5 minutes, stirring. Pour over berries, cool, and chill for half an hour.

NOTE: Kanten is a mildly diuretic sea vegetable with no calories; great for dieters. Kanten flakes may be used; figure $1/4$ to $1/3$ cup flakes equals 1 bar. Kanten may also be used to make an aspic, using vegetable or fish stock. *Makes 6–8 servings.*

FRUIT KANTEN PIE

A rich dessert—not for every day. Use any fruit with the Berry-Kanten recipe as your pie filling.

Make a simple crust by blending 2 cups whole wheat pastry flour (or other flour) and $1/2$ cup oil with your fingers. Add water to create a dough and roll out on a floured board to make one crust. Bake 10 minutes at 450 degrees. Cool. Add filling and chill half an hour or more.

PEACH HALVES

4 whole peaches, halved
and seeded
1 tablespoon lemon
juice
1 tablespoon barley malt

1 tablespoon vanilla
(optional)
1 tablespoon kanten
flakes

Stew the fruit 10–15 minutes in water to cover. Stir in lemon juice, barley malt and vanilla extract, if desired. Add kanten flakes and stir to dissolve. Arrange fruit in serving bowl and chill for half an hour before serving. *Makes 8 servings.*

FRUIT PUDDING

2 tablespoons tahini
1 cup water
3 cups apple juice
Pinch of salt
2 cups fruit, cut up
3 tablespoons kudzu

½ teaspoon vanilla
Grated lemon peel
(optional)
Chopped nuts
(optional)

Blend tahini with the water. Combine with apple juice, salt and fruit, and cook till tender. Meanwhile, dissolve kudzu in 3 tablespoons water, and add vanilla, and lemon peel, if desired. Cook over medium flame until thick and clear, and pour into individual serving dishes; chill. Garnish with chopped nuts if desired. *Makes 6–8 servings.*

QUICK FRUIT CRUNCH

2 apples, peaches or
pears

1 teaspoon kudzu
1 cup oatmeal

3 tablespoons barley
    malt or maple syrup

Pinch of salt
Cinnamon (optional)

Slice fruit and arrange in a 9-inch baking pan. Dissolve kudzu in ½ cup water. Sprinkle the oatmeal over the fruit, and pour kudzu mixture evenly over the fruit and oatmeal. Drizzle barley malt (or maple syrup) over the mixture. Sprinkle with salt and cinnamon, if desired. Bake in a 350-degree oven for 15 minutes. *Serves 2.*

NOTES: Cinnamon is not for frequent use, since it is derived from a tropical plant.

Other fruits may be used, including cherries, berries, or plums, or any mixture of these.

OATMEAL COOKIES

3 cups rolled oats
½ cup chopped nuts or
    seeds
1½ cups whole wheat
    pastry flour

Pinch of salt
2 tablespoons corn oil
¾ cup barley malt
½ cup raisins
Water or apple juice

Dry-roast the oats until slightly brown. Dry-roast the nuts or seeds (sunflower and/or sesame).

Mix flour and oats. Add salt and oil, and work through. Add malt, raisins and nuts or seeds, and mix. Add water or juice to moisten batter until it will drop from a spoon to make each cookie. Bake on a greased cookie sheet at 375 degrees for 20–25 minutes. *Makes 2 dozen.*

NOTE: For a sweeter cookie, use pure maple syrup for half of the malt.

BEVERAGES

End the meal with roasted bancha tea or grain coffee. For festive occasions, make a punch, hot or cold, of fruit juice and bancha tea. Of alcoholic beverages, beer and sake in moderation are preferred for celebrations.

For drinking water between meals, spring water is preferred. Gauge your need for liquids, and don't drink more than you need.

APPENDIX:
TABLE OF RECIPES

Recipe	Serving Suggestion	Stage
Soup as a meal		
Potage à la Bonne Femme	with hearty bread	Stage 1–2
Spinach Vichysoisse	bread and salad, Caesar salad	Stage 1–2
Meatless Minestrone	Italian bread (wine)	Stage 1–2
Genoese Minestrone	Italian bread (wine)	Stage 1–2
Lentil Mushroom	dark bread, cheese or salad	Stage 1–2
Split Pea	corn bread, salad	Stage 1–2
Barley Mushroom	hearty salad (baked squash)	Stage 1–2
Chicken Corn Chowder	salad (biscuits)	Stage 1 only

Recipe	Serving Suggestion	Stage
Mulligatawny	salad in pita pockets	Stage 1 only; adapt for Stage 2
Garden Vegetable	bread, salad	Stage 2, 1
Ukrainian Borscht	kasha pilaf, dark bread	Stage 2
Cabbage Borscht	hearty bread	Stage 2, 1
Okroshka	bread, salad	Stage 2, 1
Fish Chowder	Asparagus Vinaigrette, broccoli with cheese sauce	Stage 2, 1
Bouillabaisse	French bread, salad	Stage 2, 1
Black Bean	Greek salad, bread	Stage 2
Simple Miso	Pilaf and Bean Salad	Stage 2–3
Breakfast Miso	add leftover grain, noodles	Stage 3
Lentil	baked squash, steamed vegetables	Stage 3
Barley Mushroom	cooked greens, sourdough bread	Stage 3
Aduki Bean	baked squash, kasha	Stage 3
Black Bean	hiziki salad, kasha	Stage 3
Bonito Noodle	Boiled Green Salad	Stage 3
Onion with Fu Rounds	Boiled Green Salad	Stage 3
Hot and Sour	Boiled Rice with Corn	Stage 3
Pumpkin Soup	millet, Sesame Noodles, cooked greens	Stage 3
Watercress	baked squash, millet	Stage 3
Macrobiotic Minestrone	sourdough bread	Stage 3

Recipe	Serving Suggestion	Stage

Salad meals

Recipe	Serving Suggestion	Stage
Caesar	soup, bread or a meal in itself	Stage 1–2
Niçoise	French bread	Stage 1–2
Taco	rice and beans, lentil soup	Stage 1–2
Macaroni	sliced tomatoes, soup	Stage 2, 1
Egg	in pita pocket (soup)	Stage 2, 1
Guacamole	Taco Salad	Stage 2, 1

Entrées

Recipe	Serving Suggestion	Stage
Parmesan Chicken	Asparagus Vinaigrette, steamed potatoes	Stage 1 only
Chicken Marsala	Italian Green Beans, rice or noodles	Stage 1 only
Sesame Chicken	Snow Peas and Mushrooms, summer squash	Stage 1 only
Chicken Shish Kebab	a meal in itself (rice)	Stage 1 only
Stewed Chicken	Basic Biscuits	Stage 1 only
Chicken Paprikash	noodles, Cucumber Salad	Stage 1 only
Donna Richards's Pot Pie	a meal in itself	Stage 1 only
Chicken Parmigiana	Asparagus Vinaigrette, spaghetti	Stage 1 only
Easy Roast Chicken	potatoes, Cinnamon Carrots	Stage 1 only
Chicken Waldorf Salad	sliced tomatoes, artichokes	Stage 1 only

Recipe	Serving Suggestion	Stage
Tandoori Chicken	Cucumber Salad, Greens, Dal (Indian Side Dishes)	Stage 1 only
Steamed Fish	squash or yams, rice	Stage 1–2
Pan Poached Fish	Broccoli-Carrots-Onions, rice or potatoes	Stage 1–2
Tuna Steaks	fresh corn, tomatoes	Stage 1–2
Sea Bass with Bean Sauce	Snow Peas and Mushrooms, vermicelli noodles	Stage 1–2
Shrimp Creole	rice, salad	Stage 1–2
Paella	salad	Stage 1 only
Bluefish with Mustard Sauce	fresh corn, tomatoes	Stage 1–2
Pasta Primavera	a meal in itself	Stage 1–2
Ratatouille	salad, spaghetti	Stage 1–2
Linguine with Broccoli and Escarole	sliced tomatoes, Leftovers Vinaigrette	Stage 1–2
Fettuccine Alfredo	salad, Asparagus Vinaigrette	Stage 1–2
Linguine with Clam Sauce	salad, Italian Green Beans	Stage 1–2
Linguine with Broccoli and Scallops	sliced tomatoes, Cinnamon Carrots	Stage 1–2
Basic Marinara Sauce	spaghetti, salad	Stage 1–2
Lasagne Florentine	a meal in itself (salad)	Stage 1–2
Macaroni with Cheese	salad, steamed vegetables	Stage 1–2

Recipe	Serving Suggestion	Stage
Tuna Noodle Casserole	salad	Stage 1–2
Quick Cheddar-Squash Casserole	steamed vegetables, tomatoes	Stage 1–2
Carol's Eggplant Casserole	Fried Tomatoes, rice	Stage 1–2
Omelets	salad	Stage 1–2
Frittata	tomatoes, salad	Stage 1–2
Poached Eggs	toast, salad	Stage 1–2
Unhurried Brunch	a meal in itself	Stage 1–2
Tuna Quiche	salad, steamed vegetables	Stage 1–2
Garden Vegetable Pie	rice, salad	Stage 1–2
Stir-Fry	a meal in itself	Stage 1–2
Rice and Beans	Taco Salad	Stage 1–2
Curry	Indian Side Dishes	Stage 1–2
Shells and Broccoli	a meal in itself (tomatoes)	Stage 2, 1
Noodles Milanese	salad (Bean Salad)	Stage 2, 1
Lasagne Florentine II	a meal in itself (salad)	Stage 2
Ratatouille Tofu Lasagne	salad	Stage 2
Perfect Pesto	tomatoes, steamed vegetables	Stage 2, 1
Monkfish Newburg	Asparagus Vinaigrette, Cinnamon Carrots	Stage 2, 1
Macrotuna Casserole	salad	Stage 2
Macroroni	salad (Bean Salad)	Stage 2
Vegetable Quiche with Tofu	rice, salad	Stage 2

Recipe	Serving Suggestion	Stage
Zucchini-Feta Casserole	millet, salad	Stage 2, 1
Cheese-Lentil Loaf	millet, cooked greens	Stage 2, 1
Lentil Burgers	pita pockets, lettuce, tomato	Stage 2, 1
Tempeh Loaf	Mushroom Gravy, Cinnamon Carrots, rice	Stage 2–3
Nancy Kiessling's Eggplant	rice, salad	Stage 2, 1
Stuffed Peppers	a meal in itself (salad)	Stage 2, 1
Stuffed Winter Squash	Cooked Greens, steamed vegetables	Stage 2, 1
Almond-Cabbage Rolls	winter squash, carrots	Stage 2, 1
Wild Rice Casserole	Cooked Greens	Stage 2, 1
Beans with Rice	salad, steamed vegetables	Stage 2
Hoppin' John	Rice, Greens Southern Style (corn bread)	Stage 2
Meatless Chili	rice, salad	Stage 2
Meatless Moussaka	millet, Greek Salad	Stage 2
Skewered Tofu	Hoppin' John, Tabbouleh Salad with Millet	Stage 2
Tofu Shish Kebab	Tabbouleh Salad with Millet	Stage 2
Spanakopita	rice, Greek Salad	Stage 2
Egg Rolls	Miso Soup	Stage 2–3

Recipe	Serving Suggestion	Stage
Falafel	pita pockets with salad	Stage 2–3
Tempura	rice, salad	Stage 2–3
Broiled Tofu	Rice with Fresh Corn, Skillet Salad (for a more complete meal, add Pumpkin Soup)	Stage 3
Stuffed Squash	Boiled Green Salad (Onion Soup)	Stage 3
Tofu Stew	Pressed Salad, cooked grain (Watercress Soup)	Stage 3
Tempeh Stew	Quick Pickle, cooked grain (Watercress Soup)	Stage 3
Sushi	Boiled Vegetable Salad, Quick Pickle (Black Bean Soup)	Stage 3
Pirogi	Boiled Green Salad, Quick Pickle (Aduki Bean Soup)	Stage 3
Millet-Vegetable Casserole	Three-Bean Salad (Pumpkin Soup)	Stage 3
Cauliflower Bake	Hiziki with Carrots, cooked grain (Bonito Soup)	Stage 3
Sukiyaki	Pressed Salad, cooked grain (Aduki Bean Soup)	Stage 3
Tofu Kebab	Boiled Vegetable Salad, Rice with Fresh Corn (Simple Miso Soup)	Stage 3

Recipe	Serving Suggestion	Stage
Tofu Lasagne	Pressed Salad (Simple Miso Soup)	Stage 3
Beans with Rice	Vegetable Sauté, hiziki (Onion Soup)	Stage 3
Rice Balls	Vegetable Sauté (Hot and Sour Soup, Macrobiotic Minestrone)	Stage 3
Sesame Noodles	Boiled Green Salad, Quick Pickle (Pumpkin Soup)	Stage 3
Kasha with Vegetables	Quick Pickle, Wakame Condiment (Lentil Soup)	Stage 3
Cabbage Rolls	Boiled Vegetable Salad, Wakame Condiment (Barley Mushroom Soup)	Stage 3
Fried Rice	Boiled Green Salad, hiziki (Aduki Bean Soup)	Stage 3

RESOURCES

BOOKS

Abehsera, Michel. *Zen Macrobiotic Cooking*. New York: Avon Books, 1968.

Adams, Ruth, and Murray, Frank. *All You Should Know About Health Foods*. New York: Larchmont Books, 1975.

Casella, Dolores. *A World of Breads*. New York: David White Co., 1966.

Davis, Adelle. *Let's Eat Right to Keep Fit*. New York: Harcourt Brace Jovanovich, 1970.

Deutsch, Ronald M. *Realities of Nutrition*. Palo Alto, Calif.: Bull Publishing Co., 1976.

Dufty, William. *Sugar Blues*. Radnor, Pa.: Chilton Book Co., 1975.

Kushi, Michio. *The Book of Macrobiotics*. Tokyo: Japan Publications Inc., 1977.

Lappe, Frances Moore. *Diet for a Small Planet* (revised edition). New York: Ballantine Books, 1982.

Muramoto, Naboru. *Healing Ourselves*. New York: Swan House Publishing Co. and Avon Books, 1973.

Null, Gary, and Null, Steve. *Protein for Vegetarians.* New York: Jove Publications, 1974.

Nutrition Almanac. John D. Kirschmann, ed. New York: McGraw-Hill Book Co., Copyright 1973, 1975, 1979 by John D. Kirschmann.

Pritikin, Nathan, with McGrady, Patrick M., Jr. *The Pritikin Program for Diet and Exercise.* New York: Grosset and Dunlap, 1979.

Sattilaro, Anthony J., M.D. with Monte, Tom. *Living Well Naturally.* Boston: Houghton Mifflin Co., 1984.

————. *Recalled by Life.* Boston: Houghton Mifflin Co., 1982.

Shelton, Herbert M. *Food Combining Made Easy.* San Antonio, 1976.

————. *Superior Nutrition.* San Antonio, 1979.

Shurtleff, William, and Aoyagi, Akiko. *The Book of Tofu.* New York: Ballantine Books, 1975.

Wright, Jonathan V., M.D. *Dr. Wright's Book of Nutritional Therapy.* Emmaus, Pa.: Rodale Press, 1979.

PERIODICALS

Blair & Ketchum's *Country Journal,* Box 870, Manchester, Vt. 05254.

East-West Journal, 17 Station St., Brookline, Mass. 02147.

The Know-How Catalogue, Distribution Center C, 7 Research Park, Cornell University, Ithaca, N.Y. 14850.

The Mother Earth News, Box 70, Hendersonville, N.C. 28791.

Organic Gardening, Prevention and other Rodale publications, Rodale Press, 33 E. Minor St., Emmaus, Pa. 18049.

The Vegetarian Times, P.O. Box 570, Oak Park, Ill. 60303.

OTHER RECOMMENDED READING

Brown, Edward Espe. *Tassajara Cooking.* Boulder, Colo.: Shambala, 1973.

Case, John, and Taylor, Rosemary C.R., eds. *Co-ops, Communes and Collectives.* New York: Pantheon Books, 1979.

Clark, Linda A. *Know Your Nutrition.* New Canaan, Conn.: Keats Publishing Co., 1973.

Esko, Wendy. *Introducing Macrobiotic Cooking.* Toyko: Japan Publications Inc., 1978.

Greene, Bert. *Greene on Greens.* New York: Workman Publishing Co., 1984.

Katzen, Mollie. *The Enchanted Broccoli Forest.* Berkeley, Ca.: Ten Speed Press, 1982.

———. *Moosewood Cookbook.* Berkeley, Ca.: Ten Speed Press, 1980.

Jaffrey, Madhur. *World of the East Vegetarian Cooking.* New York: Alfred A. Knopf Inc., 1981.

Lappe, Frances Moore. *Food First: Beyond the Myth of Scarcity.* New York: Ballantine Books, 1977.

Moore, Kathleen. *The Vegetarian Times Guide to Dining in the U.S.A.* New York: Atheneum/SMI, 1980.

Robertson, Laurel; Flinders, Carol; and Godfrey, Bronwen. *Laurel's Kitchen.* New York: Bantam Books, 1976.

Sussman, Vic. *The Vegetarian Alternative.* Emmaus, Pa.: Rodale Press, 1978.

Thomas, Anna. *The Vegetarian Epicure.* New York: Random House, 1982.

Velella, Tony. *Food Co-ops for Small Groups.* New York: Workman Publishing Co., 1975.

ORGANIZATIONS

Many organizations have newsletters or periodic mailings to inform members and other readers of conferences and other news.

American Natural Hygiene Society, 12816 Race Track Rd., Tampa, Fla. 33625.

American Vegan Society, P.O. Box H, Malaga, N.J. 08328.

Common Cause, 2030 M St., N.W., Washington, D.C. 20036.

Consumers Federation, 5516 S. Cornell, Chicago, Ill. 60637.

Consumer Publications, Pueblo, Colo. 81009.

Cooperative League of the U.S.A., 1828 L St., N.W., Washington, D.C.

East-West Foundation, 17 Station St., Brookline, Mass. 02147.

Institute for Food and Development Policy, 2588 Mission St., San Francisco, Calif. 94110.

Institute for Local Self Reliance, 1717 18th St., N.W., Washington, D.C. 20009.

Kushi Institute, Box 1100, Brookline Village, Mass. 02147.

Mountain Ark Trading Co., Fayetteville, Ark., 72701 (a leading mail-order retailer of hard-to-find natural foods).

Naropa Institute, 2130 Arapahoe, Boulder, Colo. 80302.

North American Vegetarian Society, P.O. Box 72, Dolgeville, N.Y. 13329.

The Vegetarian Association of America, P.O. Box 86, Livingston, N.J. 07039.

INDEX

391

It's a dieter's dream come true!

At last! You can have the run of the supermarket— and still count calories, carbohydrates and fat— with Corinne Netzer's bestselling reference books that help you enjoy everything from mouthwatering meals to super snacks and lose weight while you're doing it!

"Perennial dieters! Weight Watchers' dropouts! This is *our* literary event of the decade!" —Gael Greene, *Life* magazine*

☐ **THE BRAND-NAME CALORIE COUNTER** (Revised and Updated)	21109-3	$4.99
☐ **THE BRAND-NAME CARBOHYDRATE** **GRAM COUNTER**	20091-1	$4.99
☐ **THE COMPLETE BOOK OF FOOD COUNTS** (Revised)	20854-8	$5.99
☐ **THE CORINNE T. NETZER** **1993 CALORIE COUNTER**	21228-6	$3.99
☐ **THE CHOLESTEROL CONTENT OF FOOD** (Revised and Updated)	20739-8	$4.50
☐ **THE CORINNE T. NETZER** **DIETER'S DIARY**	50410-4	$6.95
☐ **THE CORINNE T. NETZER FAT GRAM COUNTER**	20740-1	$4.99
☐ **THE DIETER'S CALORIE COUNTER** (3rd Edition Revised)	50321-3	$8.99

At your local bookstore or use this handy page for ordering:

DELL READERS SERVICE, DEPT. DCN
2451 South Wolf Road, Des Plaines, IL. 60018

Please send me the above title(s). I am enclosing $_____.
(Please add $2.50 per order to cover shipping and handling.) Send check or money order—no cash or C.O.D.s please.

Ms./Mrs./Mr. _____

Address _____

City/State _____ Zip _____

DCN–7/93

Prices and availability subject to change without notice. Please allow four to six weeks for delivery.